Y0-BCW-588

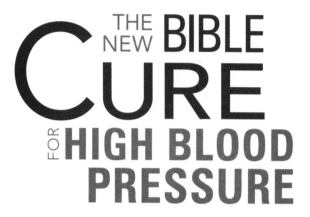

THE NEW BIBLE CURE FOR HIGH BLOOD PRESSURE

DON COLBERT, MD

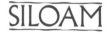

SILOAM

THE NEW BIBLE CURE FOR HIGH BLOOD PRESSURE
by Don Colbert, MD
Published by Siloam
Charisma Media/Charisma House Book Group
600 Rinehart Road
Lake Mary, Florida 32746
www.charismahouse.com

Cover design by Lisa Rae Cox and Amanda Bardwell
Design Director: Bill Johnson

Library of Congress Cataloging-in-Publication Data:
An application to register this book for cataloging has been submitted to the Library of Congress.
International Standard Book Number: 978-1-61638-615-3
E-ISBN: 978-1-62136-534-1

Portions of this book were previously published as *The Bible Cure for High Blood Pressure* by Siloam, ISBN 978-0-88419-747-8, copyright © 2001, *The Rapid Waist Reduction Diet* by Siloam, ISBN 978-1-62136-044-5, copyright © 2013, *The New Bible Cure for Cancer* by

CONTENTS

INTRODUCTION
    DISCOVER STRENGTH TO DEFEAT HIGH
    BLOOD PRESSURE ix
    A Dangerous High Blood Pressure Epidemic ix
    A Bold, New Approach x

1   UNDERSTANDING HIGH BLOOD PRESSURE 1
    How High Is Too High? 2
    A Few Tips 3
    Your Incredible Cardiovascular System 4
    With Every Beat of My Heart 6
    Wreaking Havoc on Your Arteries 6
    Causes of Hypertension 8
    Risk Factors You Cannot Control 8
        Your family history 8
        Your gender 8
        Your age 8
        Your race 9
    Secondary Causes of High Blood Pressure 9
    What Is Your Bathroom Scale Trying
    to Tell You? 10
    How Fat Is Obese? 11
    What Fruit Are You? 13
        Apple-shaped 13
        Pear-shaped 13
    Apple-Shaped Obesity 14
    The Connection Between Apple-Shaped Obesity
    (or Belly Fat) and Inflammation 14
    Conclusion 16

2   A HYPERTENSION-BUSTING DIET 18
    Slash High Blood Pressure With the DASH Diet 18

A Deadly By-Product of the Western Diet:
Inflammation 23
The Anti-Inflammatory Diet: Taking the
Mediterranean Diet to the Next Level..........................26
Conclusion..31

3 GET YOUR HEART IN SHAPE 33
Changing the Way You Think About Exercise..............33
What's in a Word? 35
The Perks of Regular Activity 36
The Natural Weight-Loss Supplement 37
Muscles, Metabolism, and Aging 38
Recommended Amount of Activity................................41
Burning Fat With Aerobic Activity 42
How Much?..44
Resistance Exercises...45
High-Intensity Interval Training 46
Putting It All Together 48
Keeping Track 48
See Your Doctor 50
Conclusion..51

4 FORTIFY YOUR HEART AND BLOOD VESSELS
THROUGH SUPPLEMENTS...53
Battling Molecular Warfare...54
Supplements to Lower Blood Pressure..........................55
   Coenzyme Q_{10}...55
   L-arginine...56
   L-citrulline...56
   Olive leaf extract 57
   Flower extracts 57
   Beetroot juice 59
Critical Minerals 60

The Power of Potassium.................................**61**

Magnificent Magnesium...............................**62**

    Are you magnesium deficient? 62

Incredible Calcium **62**

The Wonders of Water..................................**63**

    Eight glasses of water a day to help keep high blood
    pressure away 65

Hypertension Medications............................**65**

Conclusion..**66**

5   YOUR HEART AND STRESS **68**

Good Stress and Bad Stress **68**

Consequences of Stress.................................**69**

    Stress, strokes, and sickness 70

    Causes of stress.. 72

What Stress Looks Like on You **72**

Stage One: Alarm **72**

Stage Two: Resistance....................................**74**

    Gearing up to survive... 75

Stage Three: Exhaustion **76**

    When your body cannot go anymore....................... 76

Conclusion..**78**

6   COMBAT MODERN STRESS AT THE ROOT............... **80**

Activate the Power of God's Word **80**

Control Every Thought...................................**81**

Live in the Present...**81**

Tame Your Tongue...**82**

Be Quick to Forgive **83**

Get a Fresh Perspective.................................**84**

Be a Good Steward of Your Time...................**85**

Walk in the Power of Love **87**

Have a Good Laugh..**87**

Conclusion...89

7 ACTIVATE THE POWER OF DYNAMIC FAITH
   OVER YOUR HEALTH 92
   Faith for All That Concerns You.......................93
   God's Love and Your Health............................93

A PERSONAL NOTE From Don and Mary Colbert................ 95

APPENDIX A
   SUPERFOODS FOR YOUR HEART............................... 96
   Organic Celery...96
   Beetroot Juice..97
   Garlic 98
   Extra-Virgin Olive Oil 98
   Dark Chocolate 99
   Pomegranate...100
   Blueberries 101
   Wild Salmon 101
   Spinach 102
   Walnuts...102

APPENDIX B
   MERCURY LEVELS IN FOOD 103
   Fish with least amounts of mercury (enjoy these fish)....... 103
   Fish with moderate amounts of mercury (eat six
   servings or less per month) 103
   Fish high in mercury (eat three servings or less
   per month).. 104
   Fish highest in mercury (avoid)............................. 104

APPENDIX C
   SUPPLEMENTS FOR WEIGHT LOSS AND
   REDUCING HYPERTENSION 105

NOTES.. 107

DISCOVER STRENGTH TO DEFEAT HIGH BLOOD PRESSURE

G OD INTENDS TO stop high blood pressure from damaging your arteries, stressing your heart, and robbing your health. He promises to greatly strengthen your life in every way. The Bible says, "O God, You are more awesome than Your holy places. The God of Israel is He who gives strength and power to His people. Blessed be God!" (Ps. 68:35).

Do you have high blood pressure? It can be a subtle and dangerous enemy. But God promises to strengthen your heart. His Word says, "My flesh and my heart fail; but God is the strength of my heart and my portion forever" (Ps. 73:26).

If you've been told that your blood pressure is too high, then I have good news for you. You don't have to face it alone. God promises to walk with you until you defeat it. He will get you through this, and with His powerful help you will overcome it!

A DANGEROUS HIGH BLOOD PRESSURE EPIDEMIC

America is experiencing a high blood pressure epidemic. The statistics are alarming. High blood pressure—or hypertension—impacts the lives of about 68 million American adults.[1] That means that approximately one out of four people, or one in every three adults, in this country have high blood pressure.[2] The impact of all of this is alarming.

Cardiovascular disease is a killer that takes the lives of more than a million Americans every year. About half of all Americans will die of some form of cardiovascular disease. And high blood pressure is a primary reason for these deaths.

But this killer is extremely subtle and is even known as the silent killer. Most people never experience any symptoms from high blood pressure until it's advanced. So about a third of the people who have high blood pressure don't even know it! Of the people who have hypertension, only approximately 47 percent have it controlled with medication.[3]

High blood pressure triples your risk of having a heart attack. It also increases your chances of having a stroke. Forty to 90 percent of stroke victims have hypertension.[4] Strokes are the third leading killer of Americans, and they are the number one cause of long-term disability.

Among other dangers, high blood pressure can also lead to memory loss, dementia, and even Alzheimer's disease. Hypertension also damages the kidneys and may eventually lead to kidney failure.

A BOLD, NEW APPROACH

With the help of the practical and faith-inspiring wisdom contained in this Bible Cure book, you can prevent and many times overcome high blood pressure. You can usually reverse high blood pressure through the power of good nutrition, healthy lifestyle choices, exercise, vitamins and supplements, weight loss, and most importantly of all, through the power of dynamic faith.

You don't have to suffer the debilitating consequences of high blood pressure. With God's grace, health and joy await you at the end of your days!

As you read this book, prepare to win the battle against high blood pressure. This Bible Cure is filled with practical steps, hope, encouragement, and valuable information on how to develop a healthy, empowered lifestyle. In this book you will uncover God's divine plan of health for body, soul, and spirit through modern medicine, good nutrition, and the medicinal power of scripture and prayer.

You will also discover life-changing scriptures throughout this book that will strengthen and encourage you. As you read, apply, and trust God's promises, you will also uncover powerful Bible Cure prayers to help you line up your thoughts and feelings with God's plan of divine health for you—a plan that includes living victoriously.

Originally published as *The Bible Cure for High Blood Pressure* in 2001, *The New Bible Cure for High Blood Pressure* has been revised and updated with the latest medical research on this disease. If you compare it side by side with the previous edition, you'll see that it's also larger, allowing me to expand greatly upon the information provided in the previous edition and provide you with a deeper understanding of what you face and how to overcome it.

Unchanged from the previous edition are the timeless, life-changing, and healing scriptures throughout this book that will strengthen and encourage your spirit and soul. The proven principles, truths, and guidelines in these passages anchor the practical and medical insights also contained in this book. They will effectively focus your prayers, thoughts, and actions so you can step into God's plan of divine health for you—a plan that includes victory over high blood pressure.

Another change since the original *Bible Cure for High Blood Pressure* was published is that I've released a very important book, *The Seven Pillars of Health*. I encourage you to read it, because the principles of health it contains are the foundation to healthy living that will affect all areas of your life. It sets the stage for everything you will ever read in any other book I've published—including this one.

You can confidently take the natural and spiritual steps outlined in this book to combat and defeat high blood pressure forever. It is my prayer that these practical suggestions for health, nutrition, and fitness will bring wholeness to your life—body, soul, and spirit. May they deepen your fellowship with God and strengthen your ability to worship and serve Him.

—DON COLBERT, MD

A **BIBLE CURE** *Prayer for You*

Dear God, thank You for the promise of Your strength. I ask You to make me able to receive all the wisdom, strength, and power that You have for me. I thank You for strengthening my heart and restoring normal function to my arteries so that my blood pressure is normalized. Amen.

Chapter 1

UNDERSTANDING HIGH BLOOD PRESSURE

ARE YOU A wise and understanding person regarding high blood pressure? The Bible says, "Wisdom is the principal thing; therefore get wisdom. And in all your getting, get understanding" (Prov. 4:7).

According to God's Word, becoming a wise and understanding person is one of the most important things you can do. The benefits to your health and well-being cannot be measured.

> But those who wait on the LORD shall renew their strength; they shall mount up with wings like eagles, they shall run and not be weary. They shall walk and not faint.
>
> —ISAIAH 40:31

Ignorance never protects you. The Bible says the opposite is actually true. "Understanding will keep you" (Prov. 2:11). The statistics about high blood pressure may seem absolutely astonishing to you. But with wisdom and understanding, you never have to be a statistic. So let's take a careful look at high blood pressure in an effort to gain greater understanding and wisdom about it.

There are two important numbers that you need to be aware of when it comes to blood pressure. For example, if your blood pressure

1

is 120/80, the first number (120) is the systolic pressure, which is the force measured in millimeters of mercury on your arterial walls as your heart contracts to pump your blood out of the heart. Your blood pressure is at its highest when the heart beats or contracts.

The second number (80) is the diastolic pressure, which is the pressure on the walls of the arteries as your heart relaxes between beats as it is filling with blood.

A simplified analogy to understand blood pressure is to simply envision a garden hose with a nozzle on it. There are only two ways to increase the pressure in the hose. You can either turn the faucet so that maximum water flows out of the faucet, or you can tighten the nozzle on the end of the hose.

Your blood pressure usually rises the same way. If you consume too much salt or high-sodium foods, you typically retain more water, and the blood pressure rises similar to when you opened the faucet up and increased the flow of water through the hose. Excessive stress, atherosclerosis, arteriosclerosis, and endothelial dysfunction cause the arteries to constrict, like tightening the nozzle on the hose, and raise the blood pressure. If the arteries were relaxed instead of constricted, blood flow would improve and blood pressure would decrease.

HOW HIGH IS TOO HIGH?

You may be wondering, "Just how high does my blood pressure need to be in order to be considered dangerous?"

If your blood pressure is greater than 140 over 90, it's too high. But be careful; you cannot determine that you have high blood pressure based upon one elevated reading. That's unless you have a reading that is off the charts, such as an extremely high systolic blood pressure reading of 160 and a diastolic reading of 100 or higher.

Otherwise you must return to your physician's office for three different visits. At each visit your blood pressure must be measured at least twice, one or more readings on each arm. Take a look at the following chart to see how your own blood pressure ranks. These numbers are provided by the Joint National Committee on the Prevention, Detection, Evaluation, and Treatment of High Blood Pressure.[1]

A **BIBLE CURE** *Health Fact*
How Do You Rank?

You have high blood pressure if your systolic measurement is greater than or equal to 140 and your diastolic measurement is greater than or equal to 90.

Normal:
Systolic less than 120
Diastolic less than 80

Prehypertension:
Systolic 120 to 139
Diastolic 80 to 89

Hypertension, stage 1:
Systolic 140 to 159
Diastolic 90 to 99

Hypertension, stage 2:
Systolic greater than 160
Diastolic greater than 100

> He gives power to the weak, and to those who have no might He increases strength.
> —ISAIAH 40:29

A FEW TIPS

Your blood pressure rises and falls easily throughout the day. To be sure you get an accurate reading, here are a few tips to remember:

- Don't drink any coffee or caffeinated beverages for at least thirty minutes before you get your blood pressure checked.
- Don't smoke or drink any alcohol for at least thirty minutes before having your blood pressure taken.
- Sit quietly for several minutes before having your blood pressure checked.
- Talking can make your blood pressure rise, so don't talk while you are getting checked.

Here are some other factors that can influence your blood pressure:

- Diet
- Environment
- Physical activity
- Medication
- Stress
- Emotional upset

Take your blood pressure at home and keep a log of the readings.

YOUR INCREDIBLE CARDIOVASCULAR SYSTEM

Your body is an amazing creation, and your cardiovascular system is an incredible product of God's creative genius. The Bible says, "For You formed my inward parts; You covered me in my mother's womb. I will praise You, for I am fearfully and wonderfully made; marvelous are Your works, and that my soul knows very well" (Ps. 139:13–14).

Only the genius of a wonderful, divine Creator could have made you. Let's take a closer look at the amazing system of blood vessels and cells that make up your cardiovascular system.

Your cardiovascular system is composed of the heart and blood vessels. With each heartbeat, blood is released from the left ventricle into the aorta, which is a very large blood vessel that then transports the blood throughout the body. The heart is the pump, and the blood vessels are like pipes that circulate the blood.

In Deuteronomy 12:23 the Bible says that our life is in our blood, and it's really true. Your blood delivers oxygen and essential nutrients, which include vitamins, minerals, proteins, essential fats, sugars, and hormones, to all the cells in your body. The blood also removes waste products. The blood is then returned to the heart through the veins. After that it is sent to the lungs to receive a fresh supply of oxygen. And the process starts all over again.

The average pulse, which is the average heart rate, is approximately seventy beats a minute. The human heart never gets a break. It has to work continually day and night. It beats about forty-two hundred times an hour and over a hundred thousand times a day, which is over thirty-seven million times a year. When your blood pressure is normal, this presents no stress to the heart. But if your blood pressure is elevated, your heart must begin to work harder to pump the blood.

> O God, You are more awesome than Your holy places. The God of Israel is He who gives strength and power to His people. Blessed be God!
> —PSALM 68:35

WITH EVERY BEAT OF MY HEART

If your heart has to work harder with every beat, over time the left ventricle (one of the four chambers of the heart) may eventually become larger, thicker, and less compliant. It's similar to working out at a gym. When you lift weights and do curls, your muscles bulk up, becoming larger and larger. When the heart has to work harder, it actually grows larger too.

That may be great for your biceps, but it's really bad for your heart. When the size of your heart increases, it eventually leads to left ventricular hypertrophy. Let me explain what this is. As your heart gets larger, it requires more blood to nourish it. But when you have high blood pressure, your heart doesn't get the increased supply of blood it needs because high blood pressure also causes the blood vessels to become narrowed. This reduces the supply of blood to the heart.

This is why high blood pressure places you at greater risk of experiencing a heart attack and sudden death. Also, as the heart enlarges, it can become weaker since it eventually doesn't have the strength to pump effectively against the elevated blood pressure. You may then develop congestive heart failure, in which the heart becomes so weak that fluid begins to accumulate in the legs or in the lungs.

WREAKING HAVOC ON YOUR ARTERIES

High blood pressure also damages the arteries. Healthy arteries are very flexible and elastic, but high blood pressure can lead to arteriosclerosis, which is hardening of the arteries.

Here's how it works.

High blood pressure or hypertension may eventually cause atherosclerosis. In atherosclerosis the inner lining of the artery is actually damaged, usually by high blood pressure. This inner layer is the endothelium and is only one cell thick and is smooth like Teflon. The cells of the endothelium also produce nitric oxide, which dilates the arteries and also maintains the health of the endothelium. When the endothelium is damaged, platelets adhere to the site of injury, and fatty deposits begin to collect there. The once smooth, Teflon-like endothelium now becomes more like Velcro, and as fatty deposits begin to accumulate, they form plaque, which eventually hardens. The arteries become less elastic and unable to dilate adequately, which raises the blood pressure. As more damage occurs to the endothelium, it is unable to produce adequate amounts of nitric oxide to dilate the arteries, lower the blood pressure, and maintain the health of the endothelium.

The buildup of plaque can decrease blood flow even more. If the affected blood vessel is in the heart, it can lead to a heart attack. If it is in the neck or brain, it can lead to a stroke.

Continued high blood pressure can also weaken blood vessels, leading to aneurysms. An aneurysm is a weakening or bulging in the wall of an artery. An aneurysm may rupture, causing a person to bleed to death. The most common areas where aneurysms occur are in an artery in the brain and in the abdominal aorta.

A **BIBLE CURE** *Health Fact*
Sleep Apnea

Sleep apnea may eventually lead to hypertension, arrhythmias, congestive heart failure, stroke, coronary artery disease, heart attacks, cardiac arrest, pulmonary hypertension, type 2 diabetes, memory loss, and depression. One study found that one's risk of stroke doubles over a seven-year period if one has sleep apnea.[2]

CAUSES OF HYPERTENSION

There are two main types of high blood pressure: essential and secondary hypertension. About 95 percent of patients with hypertension have essential hypertension. In essential hypertension the cause is unknown. I believe that most cases of essential hypertension are caused by lifestyle, diet, obesity, excessive stress, and nutritional deficiencies. Secondary hypertension, on the other hand, is usually caused by kidney disease, medications and drugs (such as birth control pills, amphetamines, decongestants, and cocaine), and adrenal disorders. That, however, is rare, only affecting about 5 percent of people with hypertension.

RISK FACTORS YOU CANNOT CONTROL

Even though the actual cause of high blood pressure is unknown, risk factors can dramatically increase your chances of developing it. You have a great deal of control over some of these risk factors, but not all. It's impossible to have control over some risk factors. Listed below are some of them.

Your family history

If both of your parents had hypertension, there is a 60 percent chance that you will develop it. If only one parent had hypertension, you still have a 25 percent chance of developing it yourself.

Your gender

Before age fifty, men are more likely to develop hypertension. However, after age fifty, hypertension is more common in women than in men.

Your age

As you get older, your risk of developing hypertension increases.

Your race

African Americans develop hypertension twice as often as whites. Mexicans, Cubans, and Puerto Ricans are also more prone to develop hypertension.

SECONDARY CAUSES OF HIGH BLOOD PRESSURE

Secondary hypertension can be cured some of the time. Causes of secondary hypertension include kidney diseases such as polycystic kidney disease and renal artery stenosis, which is a narrowing of the arteries that supply blood to the kidneys.

Since most high blood pressure falls under the category of essential hypertension, we will focus on modifying the risk factors that we can control.

Here's a list of main risk factors:

- Medications (birth control pills, steroids, decongestants, street drugs such as cocaine and amphetamines)
- Cushing's syndrome
- Thyroid problems
- Sleep apnea (a common yet unrecognized cause)
- Obesity (especially truncal obesity)
- Pregnancy
- Kidney disease
- Inactivity
- Stress
- Lifestyle factors
- Alcohol consumption
- Smoking
- Nutritional factors

By modifying these risk factors, you should be able to control the majority of cases of mild and moderate hypertension.

Before you begin to make changes, it's very important to have a comprehensive physical exam that includes blood work, urinalysis, and an EKG. Make sure that your doctor rules out any secondary causes of hypertension.

A **BIBLE CURE** *Health Fact*

Excessive Alcohol Intake Is Associated With Hypertension

Consuming more than two servings of alcohol per day for men and more than one serving per day for women can raise blood pressure.[3]

WHAT IS YOUR BATHROOM SCALE TRYING TO TELL YOU?

How long has it been since you have weighed yourself and felt good about it? Being overweight can double your risk of developing high blood pressure. In fact, obese individuals have a two to six times greater rate of hypertension than those with normal weight. You can see why obesity is also the most important risk factor related to hypertension.

Every pound of fat in your body needs at least a mile of blood vessels to supply the fat with oxygen and nutrients. Too much blood and too many blood vessels usually lead to increased resistance within the vessels. This adds more pressure on the arterial walls, driving up blood pressure. There is usually a direct relationship between weight and high blood pressure. As your weight increases, especially in the waist, usually your blood pressure will increase also.

How Fat Is Obese?

Obesity is defined as a body mass index (BMI) of 30 or more. Body mass index is a formula that uses your weight and height to determine if your weight is normal, overweight, or obese. A BMI of 19–24.9 is healthy. A BMI of 25–29.9 is overweight, and a BMI of 30 or more is obese.

> Blessed be the LORD my Rock, who trains my hands for war, and my fingers for battle.
> —PSALM 144:1

According to federal guidelines, approximately a third of adults are overweight, and 35.7 percent are obese. Not only does obesity increase your risk of having high blood pressure, but it also increases your risk of diabetes, stroke, heart disease, and even cancer.

Hypertension is three times more common among obese patients (with BMI greater than 30) than in patients of normal weight. In more than 70 percent of patients with hypertension, the high blood pressure is directly related to obesity.

Take a look at the body mass index chart in the following Bible Cure Health Fact to determine which category—normal, overweight, or obese—you are in.

Losing weight and achieving a healthy BMI could save your life. In addition to helping you to beat high blood pressure, it will make you feel great about yourself again. Think of how wonderful it would feel to get into some of those slacks that have been pushed to the back of your closet for so long.

For natural and spiritual power to defeat obesity, read my books *The New Bible Cure for Weight Loss* and *The Rapid Waist Reduction Diet*.

A **BIBLE CURE** *Health Fact*
Body Mass Index

Too much body fat is an obvious warning sign. You can measure your body fat. Draw a line from your weight (left column) to your height (right column). Is your BMI (middle column) in the "healthy" range?

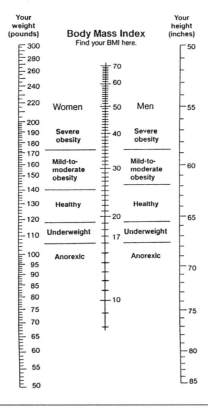

WHAT FRUIT ARE YOU?

When it comes to high blood pressure, it's not only important to understand if you're overweight, but you should also be aware of *how* you're overweight. Let me explain.

Apple-shaped

Where is your body's excess fat located? This is critically important when it comes to high blood pressure. Do you have belly fat with love handles? If you are a person with abdominal obesity, or central obesity, you are considered "apple-shaped."

If you are apple-shaped, you are much more likely to develop high blood pressure, diabetes, strokes, and coronary artery disease. The reason is this: when your fat is mainly in your abdomen, it is associated with elevated levels of C-reactive protein. CRP is a marker and a promoter of inflammation, which is the root cause of atherosclerosis or plaque buildup.

Here's how you can determine if you have an apple shape. Simply measure the narrowest area around your waist at the level of your naval and the widest area around your hips. Divide the measurement of your waist by the measurement of your hips. If this number is greater that 0.95 in men or greater than 0.8 in women, then you have an apple shape.

Pear-shaped

If your extra fat is stored in your thighs, hips, and buttocks, you are "pear-shaped." This body shape is not nearly as dangerous as apple-shaped obesity.

APPLE-SHAPED OBESITY

Many patients with apple-shaped obesity also tend to be insulin resistant. Insulin resistance is present in about half of those who have high blood pressure.

When you are insulin resistant, your cells do not properly respond to insulin. As you eat a meal with a lot of sugars or processed, refined starches, these sugars and starches break down into glucose, which is then absorbed into the bloodstream. Glucose triggers the pancreas to secrete insulin. Insulin then causes glucose and other nutrients to be delivered into the cells. As glucose enters the cells, the glucose levels in the blood fall, which then signals the pancreas to stop producing insulin.

But in many obese patients these insulin receptors in the cells do not work properly. Therefore sufficient amounts of glucose and nutrients do not reach the cells, which causes the glucose to remain in the blood. The high levels of blood glucose trigger the pancreas to continue secreting insulin. Now you have high levels of both glucose and insulin. Over time this situation usually leads to type 2 diabetes.

As insulin levels and blood sugars rise, they usually lead to elevated cholesterol and triglyceride levels, which eventually accumulate in the arteries as plaque.

THE CONNECTION BETWEEN APPLE-SHAPED OBESITY (OR BELLY FAT) AND INFLAMMATION

The obesity and inflammation connection is cyclical in nature: obesity, especially belly fat, causes increased inflammation, and increased inflammation causes more weight gain. This is partially due to fat cells manufacturing various types of inflammatory mediators, including interleukin-6, tumor necrosis factor-alpha, and plasminogen activator inhibitor-1. These all increase inflammation and are associated with atherosclerosis, or hardening of the arteries. Fat cells also produce cytokines. These are proteins that trigger the production of more inflammatory mediators, including C-reactive protein (CRP). CRP is just one inflammatory marker that doctors use to measure the body's inflammatory state. If there is inflammation anywhere in the body, CRP typically increases. The CRP level rises in cases of chronic infection, elevated blood sugar (insulin resistance), and in overweight and obese people, especially among those with increased belly fat. Elevated CRP is also associated with an increased risk of both heart attack and stroke. An elevated CRP level in turn eventually causes arteries to constrict similarly to tightening the nozzle on the hose. As belly fat increases, typically CRP increases, which triggers the arteries to constrict. Now do you get the picture and why it is so important to lose that belly fat?

When the body produces more inflammatory mediators, such as CRP, this in turn sparks chronic systemic inflammation. Essentially the more fat you have (particularly belly fat), the more inflammation you have, and we know that inflammation is the root cause of most coronary artery disease or plaque buildup in the arteries that nourish the heart. Most people think of fat tissue as inactive, but that is far from the truth. Fatty tissue or fat storage areas, such as belly fat, are active endocrine organs that produce numerous types of hormones, such as resistin (which increases insulin resistance), leptin (which decreases appetite), and adiponectin (which improves insulin sensitivity and helps to lower blood sugar). The more fat cells, the more estrogen, cortisol, and testosterone your body usually produces. This is one of the reasons obese men typically develop breasts and obese women often grow hair on their faces. Their fat cells are manufacturing more estrogen and testosterone, respectively.

When your fatty tissues spew out all these hormones—most

likely raising your estrogen, testosterone, and cortisol levels—and produce tremendous inflammation in your body, the result is weight gain. Your extra toxic belly fat then sets the stage for type 2 diabetes, heart disease, stroke, cancer, and a host of other diseases. That's because belly fat is like a wildfire. It spreads throughout your body and inflames your cardiovascular system, which eventually causes the production of inflammation and plaque in your arteries and even inflammation in the brain. This can even potentially lead to Alzheimer's disease.

In chapter 2 we will discover a hypertension-busting diet that will help you combat inflammation and belly fat.

CONCLUSION

I trust that you've gained a little wisdom and insight into what high blood pressure is and why you or your loved one has it. In the face of these medical facts your goal is to take advantage of the wealth of wisdom in God's Word and in the medical understanding with which God has blessed us. Most importantly I encourage you to take hold of the healing power of Jesus Christ that He bought for you by His own sufferings.

A **BIBLE CURE** Prayer for You

Dear Lord, thank You that You are supplying wisdom and understanding to my life. With You on my side I know I'm not a statistic. I thank You for Your love and favor in my life. I ask You for Your help to develop a new lifestyle that will free my destiny from the negative consequences of high blood pressure. Most importantly, Lord, help me to understand and to lay hold of the healing power of Jesus Christ in my life. Amen.

> For innumerable evils have surrounded me; my iniquities have overtaken me, so that I am not able to look up.
>
> —PSALM 40:12

A **BIBLE CURE** *Prescription*
Faith Builder

He was wounded for our transgressions, He was bruised for our iniquities; the chastisement for our peace was upon Him, and by His stripes we are healed.

—ISAIAH 53:5

Write out this verse and insert your own name into it: "He was wounded for _____ 's transgressions, He was bruised for _____ 's iniquities; the chastisement for _____ 's peace fell upon Him, and by His stripes _____ is healed!"

Write out a personal prayer to Jesus Christ, thanking Him for exchanging His health for your pain. Thank Him for taking the power of sickness onto His own body so that He could purchase your healing from high blood pressure.

Chapter 2

A HYPERTENSION-BUSTING DIET

Y OU ARE GOD's precious possession; His great favor is upon you. You are the apple of His eye. The Bible says, "For the LORD's portion is His people; Jacob is the place of His inheritance.... He encircled him, He instructed him, He kept him as the apple of His eye" (Deut. 32:9–10).

What a privilege it is to be chosen by God, selected by Him as the object of His love, His special care, His protection, and His guidance! You are not a statistic, destined to suffer the debilitating effects of high blood pressure. God's special love and care for you include imparting wisdom to you and healing power to help you overcome hypertension.

That wisdom includes natural nutritional solutions that can turn high blood pressure around. Let's take a look.

> They go from strength to strength; each one appears before God in Zion.
>
> —PSALM 84:7

SLASH HIGH BLOOD PRESSURE WITH THE DASH DIET

The DASH diet is a low-sodium diet especially recommended for people with hypertension or prehypertension. The letters in DASH stand for Dietary Approaches to Stop Hypertension. These are two DASH diets:[1]

1. DASH diet 1: 2,300 mg sodium/day lowers blood pressure by 11.4/5.7 mmHg (which is approximately 1 teaspoon of salt)
2. DASH diet 2: 1,500 mg sodium/day lowers blood pressure 7 to 12 mmHg

---

A BIBLE CURE *Health Fact*
High-Sodium Foods[2]

US guidelines call for less than 2,300 milligrams of sodium per day—about 1 teaspoon of table salt. And half of Americans should drop to 1,500 milligrams a day. Surprisingly, more of our salt intake is hidden in the foods we buy at the grocery store. The average American consumed 3,400 milligrams of salt a day, which is equivalent to 1½ teaspoons of salt.

Frozen dinners

They're usually loaded with sodium. A 5-ounce frozen turkey and gravy dinner can pack 787 milligrams of sodium, and most contain even more sodium.

Ready-to-eat cereals

Some brands of raisin bran have up to 250 milligrams of sodium per cup.

Vegetable juices

One cup of vegetable juice cocktail usually contains 479 milligrams of sodium.

Canned vegetables

Canned veggies are typically laden with preservatives or sauces and seasonings that add extra sodium. A cup of canned cream-style corn may contain 730 milligrams of sodium.

Packed deli meats

Beef or pork dry salami (2 slices) can pack 362 milligrams of sodium or more.

Soups

A cup of chicken noodle soup (canned) contains as much as 744 milligrams of sodium. One bouillon cube has 1,200 milligrams of sodium.

Marinades and flavorings

Teriyaki sauce (1 tablespoon) contains 690 milligrams of sodium, and soy sauce (1 tablespoon) may contain up to 1,024 milligrams of sodium.

Spaghetti sauce

Half a cup of spaghetti sauce usually packs 554 milligrams of sodium—and that amount barely coats a helping of pasta.

Cheese

Three and a half ounces of cheese typically contains 1,700 milligrams of sodium, and a medium pizza usually has much more cheese on it than 3½ ounces.

Spices

Canned jalapeno peppers (¼ cup, solids and liquids) contain about 568 milligrams of sodium.

Salted nuts

An ounce of dry-roasted, salted peanuts contains 192 milligrams of sodium.

Snack-time favorites

1-ounce serving

Potato chips = 136 milligrams

Cheese puffs = 240 milligrams

Pretzels = 385 milligrams

Even "baked" or fat-free snacks can pack the same amount of sodium or more.

Prepackaged foods

Rice, potatoes, and pasta—once you grab the convenient "all-in-one" box and add the flavor packet, you may end up eating more than half of your daily allowance of sodium in just one serving.

Pitfalls when eating out

Restaurant soups are generally very high in sodium, as are appetizers with cheeses or meats. Casserole entrées and Rice Pilaf are also common pitfalls. The word *sauce* at a restaurant is sometimes synonymous with sodium. Fish can be a lower-sodium choice at a restaurant.

Dos when eating out

Ask how food is prepared.

Choose a restaurant where food is made to order, and keep your order simple.

Ask that your meal be prepared without any form of sodium.

Studies sponsored by the National Institutes of Health have proven that the DASH diet plays a significant role in lowering blood pressure. In addition to being a low-salt (or low-sodium) plan, the DASH diet is based on an eating plan rich in fruits and vegetables, and low-fat or non-fat dairy, with whole grains. It is a high-fiber, low- to moderate-fat diet, rich in potassium, calcium, and magnesium.[3]

> The DASH eating plan has been proven to lower blood pressure in just 14 days, even without lowering sodium intake. Best response came in people whose blood pressure was only moderately high, including those with prehypertension. For people with more severe hypertension, who may not be able to eliminate medication, the DASH diet can help improve response to medication, and help lower blood pressure. The DASH diet can help lower cholesterol, and with weight loss and exercise, can reduce insulin resistance and reduce the risk of developing diabetes....
>
> New research shows that following the DASH diet over time will reduce the risk of stroke and heart disease, as well as kidney stones. The benefits of the DASH diet have also been seen in teens with hypertension.[4]

While the results of the DASH diet are well documented, I believe the best diet is the modified Mediterranean diet or the anti-inflammatory diet found in my books *The New Bible Cure for Weight Loss* and *The Rapid Waist Reduction Die*t.

The daily dietary recommendations for the DASH diet include:

- 6–12 servings of whole grains a day (However, I do not recommend grains if one has hypertension or pre-hypertension. In fact, I have found if one eliminates wheat and corn products, typically the blood pressure falls 20–40 mmHg.)
- 4–6 servings of fruit a day
- 4–6 servings of vegetables a day

- 2–4 servings of low-fat or nonfat dairy products a day

- 1½–2½ servings of lean meats, fish, or poultry a day

- 3–6 servings per week of nuts, seeds, and legumes a day

- 2–4 servings of fats and sweets[5] (I do not recommend sweets except for fruits, especially berries. I place my patients on a modified version of the Mediterranean diet or the diet I call the anti-inflammatory diet.)

Because the average American eats only about two to three servings of fruits and vegetables a day combined, some find it difficult to make the change and sustain the requirements of the DASH diet. The risks associated with not following a diet plan like the modified Mediterranean diet or the DASH diets make the whole undertaking worth the sacrifice—and the results will amaze you. Through Christ you have the power to be faithful to eating well and making healthy lifestyle choices that lead to divine health. Philippians 4:13 says that you can do all things though Christ who gives you strength.

A Deadly By-Product of the Western Diet: Inflammation

One of the biggest problems with our modern high-fat, highly processed, high-sugar, high-sodium diet is that it has thrown off the balance in our bodies between inflammatory and anti-inflammatory chemicals called *prostaglandins*. Normally inflammation is a good thing that works to repair an injury or enables you to fight off infection in the body. It puts the immune system on high alert to attack invading bacteria or viruses to rid your body of these intruders. Or in the case of an injury, it rushes white blood cells to the cut, scrape, sprain, or broken bone to splint the injury and facilitate healing. This is the good side of inflammation and an extremely important function of the immune system's small agents. When our bodies are fighting an infection, there is a complicated process through which more pro-inflammatory prostaglandins are created than anti-inflammatory ones, and the immune system responds to the sounding of this alarm. When the crisis is over, the balance swings in the anti-inflammatory direction and eventually balances out again.

A **BIBLE CURE** Health Fact
Superfoods for Your Heart

When compared to other countries, Americans have significantly more heart disease and for one reason alone: the toxic state of the standard American diet. What you eat is the single most important factor when it comes to your health. While God created many foods to nourish and protect our bodies, a few stand out when it comes to heart health and lowering the blood pressure. They include celery, beetroot, garlic, extra-virgin olive oil, dark chocolate, pomegranate, blueberries, wild salmon, spinach, and walnuts. (See Appendix A.)

But because of the high omega-6 content of our diets, and excessive sugars, processed foods, and excessive meats, our bodies produce more pro- rather than anti-inflammatory prostaglandins. Over time the natural, ongoing creation of prostaglandins will tip the balance toward systematic inflammation as more pro-inflammatory prostaglandins are produced than anti-inflammatory ones. This eventually leads to arteries constricting and the blood pressure rising. Despite the absence of an actual emergency, this imbalance still sets off alarms calling for inflammation, and the immune system will respond accordingly. This immune hypersensitivity and chronic inflammation can lead to a glut of problems ranging from simple allergies and weight gain (especially belly fat) to cancer, Alzheimer's disease, cardiovascular disease, hypertension, diabetes, arthritis, asthma, prostate problems, and autoimmune diseases.

Prostaglandins are produced from the foods we eat in an ongoing cycle, and each of the foods we eat has either a pro-inflammatory tendency or an anti-inflammatory one. Fatty acids are at the center of this. Omega-6 fatty acids are "friendly" to the creation of pro-inflammatory prostaglandins, and omega-3 fatty acids are "friendly" to the creation of anti-inflammatory prostaglandins. A more natural, Mediterranean-type diet will have a balance of pro- and anti-inflammatory-friendly foods; however, our modern high-fat, high-sodium, high-sugar, high-meat, and highly processed Western diet throws that balance off in favor of the production of pro-inflammatory prostaglandins.

Experts tell us that our typical US diet has doubled the amount of omega-6 fatty acids we consume since 1940, as we have shifted more and more away from fruits and vegetables to grain-based foods and the oils produced from them. In fact, we eat about twenty times more omega-6s than we do the anti-inflammatory omega-3 fats. Humans today consume more cereal grains—and oils produced from them—than ever before in our history, and as a result we have more inflammatory diseases—heart disease, diabetes, Alzheimer's, hypertension, and arthritis—than ever before. Most of the animals we obtain food from today are also grain fed, so most of our meats, eggs, and dairy products are higher in omega-6 fats and more inflammatory than they were a century ago. Also, as most of the fish in our stores are now farm raised, they are growing up on cereal grains instead of the algae and smaller fish they would live on in the wild, so even our fish contain more omega-6 fats than they used to. Noting all of this, it is not hard to see why diseases caused by chronic systematic inflammation have grown to be such a problem in the Western world today and especially why hypertension is an epidemic in this country.

To bring this knowledge into an individual context and see where you stand when it comes to inflammation, you can have your blood tested for C-reactive protein (CRP). CRP is simply a marker of inflammation, as well as a promoter of inflammation, and is one of the easiest indicators to test for. How high your CRP levels are will specify how significant your level of systematic inflammation is. Once you reach forty years of age, annual CRP testing is a great idea for checking the anti-inflammatory effectiveness of your diet.

Controlling inflammation is mainly done by balancing omega-6 fats and omega-3 fats through diet and supplements because these fats are not manufactured in the body. Omega-3 fat intake and the balance of different fats and oils contribute to lowering the risk of heart disease and high blood pressure. And you can do this by following the anti-inflammatory diet.

THE ANTI-INFLAMMATORY DIET: TAKING THE MEDITERRANEAN DIET TO THE NEXT LEVEL

So then, how do you escape this systemic inflammation that is causing obesity, high blood pressure, and so many health problems? First of all, you adopt the Mediterranean diet as the foundation for your day-in, day-out meal planning.

A **BIBLE CURE** Health Fact

High CRP Levels Are Not Always a Danger Sign

Although elevated CRP levels are associated with an increased risk of cancer, heart disease, diabetes, and hypertension, remember that inflammation is a natural, healthy response to disease, and any infection or injury you suffer will temporarily raise your CRP levels to fight that crisis. Avoid having your CRP levels tested for at least two weeks after you have had an acute infection or suffered an injury to ensure your serum CRP level reflects your actual consistent level and hasn't been spiked due to some recent infection.

> The Lord is my strength and song, and He has become my salvation.
>
> —PSALM 118:14

Then, within that framework, balance your pro-inflammatory and anti-inflammatory-friendly foods, and your CRP level will usually decrease accordingly. This will, of course, initially probably mean adding more anti-inflammatory foods and limiting or avoiding more pro-inflammatory ones for a time.

I highly recommend Monica Reinagel's *The Inflammation-Free Diet Plan*, where she presents her years of research to ascribe an inflammation-free (IF) rating to the foods we eat. This rating system takes into account more than twenty different factors that contribute to a food's relationship to inflammation. Positive ratings are anti-inflammatory, and foods with negative ratings promote inflammation. Up to one hundred on each scale is considered mildly one way or the other, over one hundred is moderate, and over five hundred is severe.

A **BIBLE CURE** *Health Fact*
Good-for-You Fats

All fats are not our enemy. We need to learn to choose the good fats and avoid or limit the bad, inflammatory fats. Adequate fat intake helps you maintain your protein so that your body doesn't burn protein as fuel. Fats are also the building blocks for cell membranes. Healthy fats include fatty fish, such as wild salmon; sardines; tongol tuna; anchovies; almonds; almond butter; macadamia nuts; avocados; guacamole; pecans; cashews; Brazil nuts; hazelnuts; olives; olive oil; avocado oil; macadamia nut oil; and flaxseed oil. These also include flaxseeds, chia seed, hemp seeds, and salba seeds, which are high in omega-3 fats. One may stir-fry at low heat with macadamia nut oil, olive oil, or avocado oil; but do not cook with flaxseed oil. Also, it's best to choose organic oils.

Looking at her research and adding some of my own, I have organized the following two lists of foods for you to consider adding or subtracting from your diet as your level of systemic inflammation demands.

> But He was wounded for our transgressions, He was bruised for our iniquities; the chastisement for our peace was upon Him, and by His stripes we are healed.
> —ISAIAH 53:5

DR. COLBERT'S ANTI-INFLAMMATORY DIET (ALWAYS CHOOSE ORGANIC WHEN POSSIBLE)	
Vegetables	• Steam, stir-fry, or cook under low heat. • Best cooked with extra-virgin olive oil, macadamia nut oil, or coconut oil • Vegetable soups should be non-cream-based, low sodium (homemade is best); you may add some organic meat. • Juice your own vegetable juice; avoid store-bought juices, which are usually high in sodium.
Animal proteins (meat)	• 3 oz. once or twice a day for women; 3 to 6 oz. once or twice a day for men • Wild Alaskan salmon, sardines, anchovies, tongol tuna, turkey (skin removed), free-range chicken (skin removed), eggs (pastured, organic, or omega-3 eggs as well), bison, or extra-lean beef • When grilling, slice meat into thin slices; marinate in red wine, pomegranate juice, cherry juice, or curry sauce. Remove all char from meat. • Be cautious with egg yolks, keeping to a maximum of once or twice a week. You can combine one yolk with two to three egg whites. • Limit consumption of lean beef and red meat to one to two 3 to 6 oz. servings a week.
Fruits	• Berries, Granny Smith apples, lemon, or lime. If diabetic, choose only berries.
Nuts and seeds	• All raw nuts and seeds are acceptable, but just a handful once or twice a day.
Salads	• Use 1-calorie-per-spray salad spritzers; or create your own vinaigrette spritzer using a one to two ratio of extra-virgin olive oil to balsamic, apple cider, or red wine vinegar. So you would mix 1 to 2 Tbsp. extra-virgin olive oil with 2 to 4 Tbsp. vinegar. When your body weight and waistline are normal, then increase your extra-virgin olive oil to 4 Tbsp./day and use on salads.

Dairy	• Low-fat dairy without sugar such as Greek yogurt and low-fat cottage cheese
Starches	• Sweet potatoes, new potatoes, brown/wild rice, millet bread, brown rice pasta • One to four cups daily of beans, peas, legumes, lentils, or hummus • Use moderation when choosing starches, at most only one serving per meal, and make them the size of a tennis ball, not a basketball. • If diabetic, I recommend that you avoid starches.
Beverages	• Alkaline water or sparkling water; may add lemon or lime • Green, black, or white tea; may add lemon or lime • Coffee • Low-fat coconut milk or almond milk in place of cow's milk • No sugar; use stevia or other sugar substitutes such as Just Like Sugar, Sweet Balance, xylitol, chicory, or tagatose or coconut palm sugar in moderation. • No cream; use low-fat coconut milk.
Avoid	• Avoid all gluten (wheat, barley, rye, spelt); this includes all products made with these grains, including bread, pasta, crackers, bagels, pretzels, most cereals, etc. Go to www .celiacsociety.com for gluten-free foods. • Avoid all corn products except corn on the cob that is non-GMO
Avoid	• Inflammatory animal proteins such as shellfish, pork, lamb, veal, and organ meats • Sugar • Fried foods • Processed foods • High-glycemic foods such as white rice, instant potatoes, instant oatmeal, etc.

These are not complete lists by any means—just some of the more likely "suspects" to watch out for or some of the more helpful foods to work into your diet. As you read these now, some of these will jump out at you as things you like and need, but you don't consume as much of them in your diet as you probably should. It is time to change your habits about certain foods and "lay foods on the altar" that are inviting high blood pressure into your body. The thing to remember is you have a choice about what you put in your mouth, and now that you have a little more knowledge about these foods, you can begin making healthier diet choices that will help you win the battle over high blood pressure.

I put all my patients with hypertension on a low-sodium diet and take them off all wheat and corn products as well as sugar. Renowned cardiologist Dr. William Davis takes all of his hyptensive patients off all wheat and corn products and typically sees a 20–40 mm mercury drop in their blood pressure. Please read my book *What Would Jesus Eat?*, which is the Mediterranean diet, but leave off the wheat and corn.

CONCLUSION

Changing the way you eat can be the most difficult thing you ever do. But you're not alone. Never forget that regardless of where you are on your health transformation journey, God loves you and you are still the apple of God's eye. He is ready and eager to give you the help you need to live a healthier, more joyful life. Choose to take Him at His Word. You won't be sorry!

A **BIBLE CURE** Prayer for You

Dear Jesus, I make up my mind right now to choose to believe Your Word. I may not understand why, but Your Word says that You love me deeply, and despite my weaknesses and imperfections, I'm still the apple of Your eye. With Your help day in and day out, I will change my eating habits to ones that honor You, protect my health, and lower my blood pressure. In Jesus's name, amen.

A **BIBLE CURE** Prescription
Keep a Daily Food Diary

Date/ Weight	Breakfast	Snack	Lunch	Snack	Dinner
/					
/					
/					
/					
/					
/					
/					

Chapter 3

GET YOUR HEART IN SHAPE

WHETHER YOU REALIZE it or not, you are a very privileged character. God not only sees you as an object of His love, but He also created you as the object of His special care. Here is another Bible verse that speaks of you as especially chosen by God: "He who touches you touches the apple of His eye" (Zech. 2:8).

What a wonderful privilege it is to know and recognize His amazing love and incredible care! He created you to be truly unique—one of a kind. And not only did He grace you with your life, but He also blessed your life with purpose. He will help you to understand and obtain the destiny He has for you.

Although diseases such as high blood pressure might try to get in the way of your destiny, it's also God's will to help you to overcome.

Developing a healthier lifestyle will help, and regular exercise, a natural remedy for high blood pressure, is an important part of that lifestyle. Let's examine the role of exercise and lifestyle changes in helping you to live in the destiny of favor that God has for you.

CHANGING THE WAY YOU THINK ABOUT EXERCISE

If you hate working out, you are not alone. Even big-name celebrities who are known for their ultra-fit bodies and sex appeal disdain it. Singer and actress Janet Jackson says, "I hate working out—and hate is a strong word, but I cannot stand working out."[1] Bruce Willis, known for his tough-guy roles in numerous action-adventure flicks, admits, "I'm lazy, I hate working out, I only do it for films and I think of it as work."[2]

Nor is Willis the only Hollywood star with an aversion to exercise. Actress Katherine Heigl, best known for her Emmy Award–winning performances on *Grey's Anatomy*, says, "If I wasn't in this industry, I wouldn't work out. But I have hips and a butt and everything that goes along with that, including cellulite."[3]

From the world of athletics, listen to tennis star Serena Williams: "I hate working out more than anything, but I have to—when I'm running, I think about how much I want to win. That's the only thing that keeps me going....I guess everyone has to find that one thing that encourages them and just think about it the entire time you're working out. But I have to be honest, I hate going to the gym. I don't like running. I hate doing anything that has to do with working out."[4]

The one person you might have expected to champion exercise was fitness buff Jack LaLanne, who died in January of 2011 at age ninety-six. Even the legendary workout master once said, "I hate exercise, but I love the results."[5] Such quips illustrate our love-hate relationship with exercise. In particular we dread taking the time out of our already cramped schedules for it. What other explanation is there for all the late-night TV infomercials about time-saving exercise gadgets promising pounds will "instantly" fall off if we use their product? We always want the quick solution.

As a result, two-thirds of all Americans are not physically active on a regular basis. Less than half get less than the recommended amount of exercise. Sadly a full 25 percent—a quarter of the population!—get absolutely no exercise.[6] The leading reason, according to almost every survey conducted, places time at the top of its list of excuses.[7] People rationalize they are just too busy to exercise. According to the CDC, the average adult, age eighteen to sixty-four, needs 150 minutes (2.5 hours) a week of moderate aerobic activity and two or more days a week of muscle-strengthening activity.[8] A recent study found that women over forty-five years of age need 60 minutes of moderate exercise a day to prevent weight gain as they aged, even with consuming a normal diet.[9]

WHAT'S IN A WORD?

For many the word *exercise* conjures up the same negative feelings as *diet*. Those who are overweight or obese think of exercise in terms of pain, sweating, humiliation, embarrassment, and anxiety. They may visualize themselves in a health club surrounded by people with perfect bodies, a physical education instructor testing their lack of physical capabilities, or an overbearing coach from their youth. Because this word often stimulates dread, I use a different one: *activity*. To some this seems a bit silly. It's just a word, after all—what difference could substituting one word make? Isn't it still referring to the same thing?

I cannot explain why this works, but it does. *Activity* seems less intrusive; it doesn't trigger emotional symptoms or anxiety. For most overweight or obese individuals it is safe and nonthreatening. It does not overwhelm them with thoughts of time commitments, discipline, or early-morning alarm clocks.

It is up to you whether you adapt a change of vocabulary. However, the bigger issue you cannot overlook is that both a change of diet and regular activity are crucial for weight loss. Plain and simple the reason why people successfully lose weight and keep it off is because they are physically active.

THE PERKS OF REGULAR ACTIVITY

In case you need a reminder, here are some of the many benefits that come with regular activity:

- It decreases the risk of heart disease, stroke, and the development of hypertension.
- It helps prevent type 2 diabetes.
- It helps protect you from developing certain types of cancer.
- It helps prevent osteoporosis and aids in maintaining healthy bones.
- It helps prevent arthritis and aids in maintaining healthy joints.
- It slows down the overall aging process.
- It improves your mood and reduces the symptoms of anxiety and depression.
- It increases energy and mental alertness.
- It improves digestion.
- It gives you more restful sleep.
- It helps prevent colds and flu.
- It alleviates pain.
- And the favorite reason among overweight and obese people...it promotes weight loss and decreases appetite.

Don't use Hollywood stars or fitness gurus as an excuse to justify a lack of activity. When push comes to shove, you must do your part and get moving regularly. This takes courage. If it didn't, everyone would do it. You must take the offensive to battle, remembering that obesity is a scourge that can weaken and damage other organs in your body.

THE NATURAL WEIGHT-LOSS SUPPLEMENT

There is no better way to complement a weight-loss dietary and supplement program than physical activity. How does it help? The ways are as plentiful as the many benefits I just listed. First, it helps raise the metabolic rate during and after the activity. It enables you to develop more muscle, which raises the metabolic rate all day—even while you sleep. It decreases body fat and improves your ability to cope with stress by lowering the stress hormone cortisol.

Such activity also raises serotonin levels, which helps reduce cravings for sweets and carbohydrates. It assists in burning off dangerous belly fat and improves your body's ability to handle sugar. Finally, regular physical activity can even help control your appetite by boosting serotonin levels, lowering cortisol, and decreasing insulin levels (which can also decrease your chances for insulin resistance).

There are numerous enjoyable activities to choose from; for example, cycling, swimming, working out on an elliptical machine, dancing, and hiking. Sports such as basketball, volleyball, soccer, football, racquetball, tennis, and squash are all considered aerobic. Pilates, ballroom dancing, washing the car by hand, working in your yard, and mowing the grass qualify too—anything that raises the heart rate enough to burn fat.

A great aerobic activity is brisk walking, although for diabetic patients with foot ulcers or numbness in the feet, walking is not the best activity. In its place they should try cycling, an elliptical machine, or pool activities while inspecting the feet before and after activity.

If you can walk, to enter your target heart rate zone, walk briskly enough so that you cannot sing and slowly enough so that you can talk. Following this formula is one reason that I recommend people find an activity partner to talk with them as they walk. (Skeptics might say that misery loves company.) Here are a few other tips to get you started:

- Choose something that is fun and enjoyable. You will never stick to any activity program if you dread or hate it.
- Wear comfortable, well-fitting shoes and socks.
- If you are a type 1 diabetic, you will need to work with your doctor in order to adjust insulin doses while increasing your activity. Realize that exercising will lower your blood sugar; this can be potentially dangerous in a type 1 diabetic.

MUSCLES, METABOLISM, AND AGING

Everyone wants to look young and fit forever. That's particularly true in the United States, where we plaster buff, sculpted, trimmed, toned, and youthful bodies all over magazine covers, TV ads, and movie screens. Great looks hide the reality that adults typically lose ½ to 1 pound of muscle tissue every year after the age of twenty-five, meaning our bodies naturally progress toward more fat and less muscle. That isn't the greatest news for those overloaded with fat. However, such a realization can be a driving force to shape up. The more muscle mass, generally the higher your metabolic rate and the more calories you will burn at rest. For each pound of muscle mass that you either gain or do not lose, you will burn between thirty and fifty calories a day.

A **BIBLE CURE** *Health Fact*

Chiropractic Adjustment to C1 Vertebra Lowers Blood Pressure

A study shows that a chiropractic adjustment to the C1 vertebra, also known as the "atlas adjustment," lowers systolic blood pressure by an average of 14 mmHg and an average of 8 mmHg for diastolic blood pressure.[10]

I will never forget the patient I saw years ago during residency. The star running back on a high school football team, he had fractured his left thigh. Part of the reason he played running back was the power in his legs. Not surprisingly his thighs were extremely muscular. Before, he said, he had been able to leg press more than a thousand pounds for ten repetitions. Because of his injury, though, this athlete had to wear a full leg cast for approximately two months.

When we removed the cast, we were shocked at how much his left leg had atrophied. Measuring his thighs showed a 32-inch circumference around his mid-right thigh; his left checked in at a mere 24 inches. In only two months inactivity had cost this young man 8 inches of muscle.

A similar process occurs with most adults, though not as

quickly. Yet if you are inactive, your muscles are slowly melting away. Your metabolic rate is decreasing, and muscle tissue is (typically) being replaced with fat. Many people do not notice because the size of their arm or leg remains the same, when in fact it is simply a case of fat replacing muscle tissue—similar to the marbling of meat.

This is particularly true for women. A woman's metabolism typically begins to decrease at age twenty at a rate of about 5 percent per decade. To understand this, let's use the example of an average fifty-year-old female—I'll call her Sarah. Since her late twenties Sarah's weight has slowly increased from around 120 pounds to her current weight of 150. During those years she gained 30 pounds of fat while losing 15 to 30 pounds of muscle. That may sound like it averages out, except when you consider the corresponding drop in metabolic rate.

At twenty Sarah could eat 2,000 calories a day and maintain her 120-pound frame. At the age of fifty if she eats 2,000 calories a day, she will most likely gain weight because of this lost muscle tissue. Why? For each pound of muscle tissue lost, your metabolic rate decreases 30 to 50 calories per day. So in addition to losing fifteen pounds of muscle, Sarah lost the ability to burn 450 to 750 more calories a day.

Can you see why maintaining or gaining muscle mass is so crucial? Muscle does not just look better than fat; it is essential for maintaining a healthy body. The only way to keep muscle intact is to use it and strengthen it, which means increasing your activity level. When you remain inactive, you put yourself in a body cast— so to speak—as your metabolic rate nosedives and you slowly morph into a fat magnet.

RECOMMENDED AMOUNT OF ACTIVITY

Once I have persuaded patients they need more activity, their next question is: "How much do I need?" Unfortunately no universal number applies. The Centers for Disease Control and Prevention (CDC) recommends one hundred fifty minutes of moderate intensity activity such as brisk walking a week. This translates into thirty minutes a day, five days a week. There are numerous factors involved in engaging in activity to lose weight, starting with the heart.

Every activity either requires or can be performed at different levels of intensity. Given that, it makes sense that every person hoping to lose weight has an ideal intensity at which he or she should work out. This is called your target heart rate zone, which generally ranges from 65 to 85 percent of your maximum heart rate.

To calculate the low end of this zone, start by subtracting your age from 220. This is your maximum heart rate. For example, for someone forty years old the formula is:

220 - 40 = 180 beats per minute

Multiply this number by 65 percent to find the low end of the target heart rate zone:

180 x 0.65 = 117 beats per minute

To figure out the high end of the zone, multiply maximum heart rate by 85 percent, or:

180 x 0.85 = 153 beats per minute

So, if you are forty, you should keep your heart rate between 117 and 153 beats per minute when exercising. However, that is quite a wide range, which prompts the next question: which end of the zone do you aim for to lose weight? Experts have debated this ever since the "target zone" idea came into being many years ago. To find the answer, let's look at the types of activity that push the heart to these two extremes.

BURNING FAT WITH AEROBIC ACTIVITY

The word *aerobic* means "in the presence of air or oxygen." Aerobic activity is simply movement that strengthens the lungs and the heart. It involves steady, continuous movements that work large muscle groups in repetitive motion for at least twenty minutes. The key point for weight loss with aerobic activity is to maintain a moderate pace, which triggers your body to burn fat as its preferred fuel.

One of the most common workout mistakes I see among overweight people is their tendency to jump on a treadmill and run as hard as they can for as long as possible. They intend to burn off more fat by doing this, but in the long run (pardon my pun) they won't. Sprinting, running, or jogging at high intensity for so long you are short of breath actually makes you burn less fat as fuel.

For inactive individuals who are just starting to work out, it's also the quickest way to burnout.

Remember, *aerobic* means with oxygen; therefore, the activity you choose must be of moderate intensity for your body to use oxygen in order to burn the fat as fuel. When you exercise to the point that you are severely short of breath, you are no longer performing aerobically. Instead you have shifted to an anaerobic activity, which means activity without oxygen. Anaerobic activity burns glycogen—stored sugar—as primary fuel instead of fat.

When you run out of glycogen and have not eaten for a while, you may begin breaking down muscle tissue and burning muscle protein as fuel. (Notice that I haven't yet mentioned burning fat.) Many marathoners and triathletes burn a significant amount of muscle as fuel, which is often why they remain so lean.

If you are overweight and aim to burn primarily fat, you need to work out at a moderate intensity of 65 to 75 percent of your maximum heart rate. This is the fat-burning range of your target heart rate zone. As you approach the high end, you near anaerobic activity, which does less good in burning fat. This might be a completely revolutionary idea. If so, it may be a struggle to change. Most people believe that to the hardest worker—meaning the guy who runs the fastest and sweats the most—go the spoils. Not true. If you are overweight or obese, working out at a higher intensity for long stretches may not only sabotage your fat-burning ability, but it may also increase cortisol levels, which can cause more belly fat to accumulate.

When starting any activity program, work out around 65 percent of your maximum heart rate. As you become more aerobically conditioned, gradually increase the intensity to 70 percent of your maximum heart rate. After a few more weeks increase to 75 percent, and so on. You may never be able to work out at 85 percent of maximum rate, especially if you are huffing and puffing. The best fat-burning zone is usually 65 to 75 percent of your maximum heart rate. Be sure that as you increase the intensity of your workouts, you remain able to converse with another person. That is a fairly good sign that you are training aerobically and are burning fat. When you are in good aerobic condition, you can start interval training.

HOW MUCH?

This brings us back to the original question: how much activity? The CDC and the National Institutes of Health (NIH) both recommend following the *2008 Physical Activity Guidelines for Americans*, published by the US Department of Health and Human Services. The guidelines recommend that adults need two types of physical activity each week—aerobic and muscle-strengthening. For aerobic activity they recommend two hours and thirty minutes of moderate intensity aerobic activity a week or thirty minutes of moderate exercise five days a week (brisk walking, water aerobics, riding a bike on level ground, playing doubles tennis, pushing a lawn mower, etc.) or one hour and fifteen minutes of vigorous exercise or twenty-five minutes of vigorous exercise three days a week (jogging, swimming laps, riding a bike fast or on hills/inclines, playing singles tennis, playing basketball, etc.). For muscle-strengthening exercise, which I call resistance exercise, they recommend two or more days a week, working all major muscle groups (legs, hips, back, abdomen, chest, shoulders, and arms).[11]

I recommend breaking up the aerobic activity as follows: if you can only do moderate intensity activities, try brisk walking for thirty minutes a day, five days a week. If you can handle more vigorous activity, jog for twenty-five minutes a day, three days a week. Or you can break it down even further: try going for a fifteen-minute walk, two times a day, five days a week.

Clearly it pays to be active. The longer you engage in activity at a moderate intensity, the more fat you burn as fuel. I am not suggesting you have to jog twenty miles a week. Still, you can start by choosing enjoyable, fun activities that you and your family can do daily to obtain similar results. Unless you have already been working out, I suggest that you initially set a goal of twenty minutes a day, which may be split into ten minutes, twice a day. (You can do this by simply walking your dog!) Once you have adapted, gradually increase to thirty minutes and eventually forty minutes or more.

To minimize soreness, get activity every other day, three days a week, and work up to five or six days a week. And remember, a brisk walk can accomplish almost as much as jogging—provided you maintain 65 to 75 percent of your maximum heart rate.

RESISTANCE EXERCISES

Resistance training usually involves lifting weights to build muscles. These strengthening activities include weight training with free weights or machines, calisthenics, Pilates, resistance band activities, core-specific activities, and balance ball activities. To eliminate the risk of injury, you must maintain good posture and form while performing these exercises. In addition it is important to learn the correct lifting techniques, the correct range of motion, correct breathing, and the correct speed of the movement in which muscles are being trained. It is very important to not hold your breath while lifting since this can raise your blood pressure. Also do not lift heavy weights since the straining may also raise your blood pressure. Simply do ten repetitions with moderate weight for each exercise, and be sure to breathe correctly with each repetition.

You should typically perform ten to twelve repetitions per set. When starting resistance training, I recommend only performing one set per activity. This reduces soreness, which is common in beginning any type of strengthening program. As you become better conditioned over time, you can increase to two or three sets per activity for each body part to strengthen and tone muscles.

Remember, go slow! Strength training causes microscopic tears in muscle fibers, which eventually causes them to grow stronger and larger. This in turn increases your metabolic rate. Never overdo it and train the same muscles every day; the muscles will not have time to repair and rebuild.

> A wise man is strong, yes, a man of knowledge increases strength.
> —PROVERBS 24:5

Eventually, after a few weeks of strength training, you may be able to increase your workouts to three or four days a week. By following the correct lifting techniques, you will prevent injury, build muscle, and burn fat. I recommend finding a certified personal trainer to teach you this valuable information so you can maximize results. After years of visiting health clubs, I am appalled at the large percentage of people who lift weights incorrectly. I discuss this in more detail in my book *Get Fit and Live!*

HIGH-INTENSITY INTERVAL TRAINING

If you've had any success in the past with high-intensity workouts, my guess is that the past few pages of this chapter may have frustrated you. It's hard to convince avid weightlifters and spinning aficionados that moderate-intensity workouts are the best way to burn fat. Most everyone has been trained that the harder you work out and the more you sweat, the more fat you shed. I've already discussed the reasoning for my moderate-intensity preference, but let me explain this a little further before going on.

High-intensity anaerobic workouts obviously have proven value.

Not only that, but also studies in recent years have shown that these power cardio routines can be just as effective as longer, moderate-intensity workouts.

It's no surprise, then, that the American public, with its usual "faster is better" mind-set, has adopted this as the preferred way to lose fat. However, after helping thousands of overweight and obese individuals to successfully lose weight and keep it off, I believe I have enough credentials to speak on this matter. Let me offer a suggestion for those who have exercised religiously in the past or who become bored quickly with moderate-intensity workouts. Try varying it up once in a while with some high-intensity interval training (HIIT). Notice the word *interval*, however. This is simply alternating between brief, hard bursts of exercise and short stretches of lower-intensity exercise or rest. Various studies in recent years have proven this to be an effective way to improve not only overall cardiovascular health but also your ability to burn fat faster. One study at the University of Guelph in Ontario, Canada, found that following an interval training session with an hour of moderate cycling increased the amount of fat burned by 36 percent.[12]

I personally do HIIT three times a week. I warm up on the elliptical machine for five to ten minutes. I then do sixty seconds of high-intensity training with high resistance and as fast as I can. I then decrease the resistance and speed to a lower setting so that I can talk while exercising for sixty seconds. I continue this pattern for twenty to thirty minutes.

My suggestion is to hold off on HIIT, regardless of your exercise past, until you've consistently done some moderate-intensity activity for several months. I'd rather see you be able to sustain your momentum for the long haul rather than have you burn out, not because of eating the wrong things, but simply because you wanted to sprint to the finish line faster. Be sure to have a physical exam with EKG and or a stress test before starting HIIT.

A **BIBLE CURE** *Health Tip*
The Tabata Method

A popular new form of HIIT is Tabata, an exercise regimen created by Izumi Tabata that uses twenty seconds of high-intensity exercise followed by ten seconds of rest, repeated for eight cycles. An alternative routine uses three minutes of warming up, followed by sixty seconds of high-intensity exercise, followed by seventy-five seconds of rest, repeated for eight to twelve cycles.

PUTTING IT ALL TOGETHER

To lose weight, you can literally start your activity program on the right foot. Unless you are physically restricted, walking is the easiest way to stay active. All you need for equipment are some comfortable clothes and a good pair of walking shoes. It's a great way to enjoy the outdoors. Follow my earlier recommendation to find an activity partner, and you can catch up on conversation while he or she holds you accountable with your exercise. Avoid the routine; for variety, go to a park or visit a hiking trail.

KEEPING TRACK

Researchers say that self-monitoring devices, such as a pedometer, heart rate monitor, or even a simple exercise journal can account for a 25 percent increase in successfully controlling your weight.[13]

I believe in monitoring yourself. An excellent way to monitor the steps you walk during the day is by using a pedometer. I urge all my patients to get one and track their step count during the day. Typically a person walks three thousand to five thousand steps a day. To stay fit, set a goal of ten thousand steps, or approximately five miles. To lose weight, aim for between twelve thousand and fifteen thousand steps per day. Other ways to reach this upper target: walking your dog, parking farther out in the parking lot at work or when shopping, and taking the stairs instead of the elevator whenever possible.

Before engaging in any activity, make sure that you have either eaten a meal two or three hours prior or have had a healthy snack about thirty to sixty minutes beforehand. It is never good to work out when hungry; you may end up burning muscle protein as energy—which is very expensive fuel. Remember, losing muscle lowers your metabolic rate.

After you are into the routine of walking approximately thirty minutes, five or six days a week, or you are taking twelve thousand steps a day on your pedometer, you can start resistance training. Before this routine, always do a five-minute warm-up by walking on a treadmill or elliptical machine or riding a stationary bike at low intensity. This increases blood flow to muscles and joints, prepares them for the workout, and significantly reduces the risk of injury.

Once you have warmed up, do a twenty- to thirty-minute workout, using free weights, machines, calisthenics, Pilates, or some other strengthening activity. This burns up much of the glycogen stored in the muscles and liver. Following this, you will be ready for a thirty-minute aerobic workout, such as brisk walking on a treadmill, cycling, or using an elliptical machine or other cardio equipment. This aerobic session allows you to mainly burn fat. When you are finished with both the strength and aerobic parts of your workout, cool down by doing a low-intensity aerobic activity for another five minutes—just as you warmed up. You may also want to do some stretching after your cooldown.

I recommend a resistance program two to four days a week, working out every other day for twenty to thirty minutes, and an aerobic program five to six days each week for thirty minutes. Always warm up before any activity and cool down at the end. And keep things fun by periodically changing the routine. By varying your activities every month or so, you can shock your muscles into new growth—which means burning more fat. That is a step everyone should want to take. A simple way to maximize fat burning is to take a thirty-minute walk in the morning before eating breakfast. Simply drink 12–16 ounces of water and go for a brisk walk. You see, during the night you probably have burned off most of your glycogen (stored sugar) stores in your liver and muscles. By walking in the morning before breakfast, you will be burning mainly fat and the blood pressure usually gradually decreases.

SEE YOUR DOCTOR

If you have multiple cardiovascular risk factors such as hypertension, a smoking history, high cholesterol, or a strong family history of heart disease, I strongly recommend that you get a physical examination and undergo an exercise stress test before beginning an exercise program.

Every year in the United States about seventy-five thousand Americans have a heart attack during or after vigorous exercise. These are generally people with a sedentary lifestyle or who have risk factors for heart attack. Even after your physician has medically cleared you for exercise, avoid intense exercise until your cardiovascular risk factors have been modified and your cardiovascular fitness has improved.

Individuals living in northern states generally experience more incidents of heart attack while shoveling snow after heavy snow falls. But if you are young with mild hypertension and exercise moderately, your risk for heart attack is extremely low. In fact, researchers have found that fewer than ten individuals out of one hundred thousand will have a heart attack during exercise. Those who do suffer heart attacks are usually sedentary with other risk factors for heart disease, and they exercise too hard for their level of fitness.

If you experience tightness in the chest while exercising, chest pain or pain down the left arm or up into the jaw, rapid heartbeats, light-headedness, or severe shortness of breath, seek medical attention immediately. In addition, I strongly advise against exercising near heavy traffic since the carbon monoxide and air pollution are toxic and can damage the heart and blood vessels.

Conclusion

Becoming a more active person will not only lower your blood pressure and protect your heart, but as you develop a healthier and more active lifestyle, you will also discover many other powerful benefits. You will begin to feel better physically, mentally, and emotionally. You will also begin to look better as you begin to lose weight and tone your muscles.

As you get started, remember that God is with you to help you. Whisper a prayer to Him for help whenever you need it. He will help you to stay motivated and keep at it. You will begin to experience the joy and excitement of your destiny as one who is highly favored by God as the apple of His eye!

A **BIBLE CURE** Prayer for You

Dear Lord, thank You for Your wonderful favor upon my life. Thank You that my life is more valuable to You than it is to me, and that You have made me the apple of Your eye. Thank You for planning a destiny for me that includes good health and a long, productive, and blessed life. Help me to begin a new lifestyle of regular exercise and activity. Help me to be faithful and disciplined. In Jesus's name, amen.

A **BIBLE CURE** Prescription

Make note in your journal of the lifestyle changes you plan to make:

❏ Exercise regularly.

❏ I plan to begin a program of _____.

❏ Begin an aerobic program.

❏ Purchase fitness equipment for my home.

❏ Begin ballroom dancing or _____ .

❏ Begin parking my car at the back of the lot or _____ .

Write your own prayer in your journal asking God for help in making these lifestyle changes.

_____

_____

Then write a prayer of commitment asking God for His help in staying faithful to an exercise program.

_____

_____

Chapter 4

FORTIFY YOUR HEART AND BLOOD VESSELS THROUGH SUPPLEMENTS

A S PART OF God's great love and favor in your life, He has graced the world with everything you need to be healthy. The Bible says, "He causes the grass to grow for the cattle, and vegetation for the service of man, that he may bring forth food from the earth" (Ps. 104:14).

God has provided what your body needs to be healthy and fit. But too often our hectic eating habits, poor food choices, and nutrient-depleted foods rob our bodies of the benefits God intended. Even so God has still made provision for us, for He has promised to supply all of our needs. The Bible says, "My God shall supply all your need" (Phil. 4:19). God is well aware of the time and circumstances in which we live, and in His great love for us He has provided for our care.

You may be thinking, "But how does this relate to supplements? Aren't these made by man?" They are, but the knowledge and understanding, as well as the materials, are all given by God. The Word of God says, "The earth is the LORD's, and all its fullness. The world and those who dwell therein" (Ps. 24:1).

Even though much of the food we eat doesn't totally supply the vitamin and mineral requirements of our bodies, God has graced our world with the know-how to make up the lack. And when it comes to high blood pressure, supplements can make all the difference in the world.

Let's take a look at some supplements that are an essential part of your Bible cure for high blood pressure.

BATTLING MOLECULAR WARFARE

Taking supplements can greatly strengthen your body's ability to battle the devastating effects of free radicals. You probably don't realize it, but right now your cells are fighting a molecular atomic war. At this very moment free radicals are bombarding your body, creating molecular havoc. Let me explain.

Free radicals are unstable molecules that damage healthy cells like a kind of molecular shrapnel, creating chain reactions of cellular destruction. Free radicals cause oxidation. When metals such as iron are oxidized, rust is produced. When you cut an apple in half, it begins to turn brown within a few minutes due to oxidation. Free radicals are generated in our bodies simply by breathing. Normal metabolism creates free radicals referred to as reactive oxygen species. Certain types of food will create excessive free radicals, including hydrogenated, partially hydrogenated, and trans fats; deep-fried and pan-fried foods; excessive polyunsaturated fats, which are usually present in salad dressings; excessive sugar and processed foods; and excessive intake of red meat and processed meats. Smoking, exposure to pollution, and inflammation all increase free radicals. Free-radical damage also contributes to hypertension and atherosclerosis.

When high blood pressure goes untreated for too long, your arteries lose their elasticity and actually begin to form plaque. The hypertension causes shearing forces that injure the lining of the arterial walls, causing the buildup of even more plaque. More and more plaque builds up until arteries eventually become blocked or the plaque ruptures forming a blood clot causing a heart attack.

That's why antioxidants are critically important. Like Patriot missiles, they quench many of these free-radical reactions and protect the lining of the blood vessels from further plaque buildup. Let's look at some of these powerful defenders.

SUPPLEMENTS TO LOWER BLOOD PRESSURE

Coenzyme Q_{10}

Coenzyme Q_{10} (CoQ_{10}) has several benefits for the cardiovascular system that help lower blood pressure and normalize heart contraction and rhythm. It also helps improve energy production at the cellular level by improving mitochondrial function. The mitochondria are like tiny energy factories inside each cell. Heart muscle cells have the most mitochondria because they never stop working and fat cells have the least mitochondria. Individuals with hypertension, or high blood pressure, are often deficient in coenzyme Q_{10}.

Coenzyme Q_{10} is found in foods such as fish, especially sardines and mackerel. (See Appendix B regarding the mercury levels in these fish.) It can also be found in peanuts, soy oil, whole-grain germs, and organ meats such as heart, liver, and kidney, as well as beef (but use caution with consuming these meats).

Research has shown that coenzyme Q_{10} reduces blood pressure. In one study subjects experienced significantly improved systolic and diastolic pressure and an overall improvement of heart function. Some were able to completely stop their blood pressure medication four months after starting supplementation with coenzyme Q_{10}.

As we age, CoQ_{10} levels decline, so older persons should always be checked out to determine potential CoQ_{10} deficiency. I commonly check CoQ_{10} blood levels on elderly patients with heart disease. Certain medications used for cardiovascular conditions actually deplete the body of coenzyme Q_{10}: thiazide diuretics, beta blockers, clonidine, methyldopa, and especially cholesterol-lowering agents such as statin medications (statin) and fenofibrates.[1]

I recommend the active form of CoQ_{10} (ubigquinol) 100 milligrams two times a day. (See Appendix C.)

L-arginine

L-arginine is an amino acid that improves blood flow and improves the activity of the endothelial cells. Endothelial cells or the endothelium is the layer of cells that line the interior surface of blood vessels and is very thin, only one cell thick, and very fragile. When the endothelium is well nourished, optimal amounts of nitric oxide is produced by these cells. Nitric oxide, or NO, helps maintain the elasticity of all blood vessels and especially the arteries. NO is also a signaling molecule that signals arteries to dilate, which helps to lower one's blood pressure. L-arginine is converted to NO in the body; however, one cannot consume adequate amounts of L-arginine from food alone. Arginine is present in red meat, chicken, fish, soy nuts, beans, and dairy.

The typical dose of L-arginine to lower blood pressure is 2 to 3 grams or more twice a day, in the morning and at bed time. (See Appendix C.)

L-citrulline

This is another amino acid that is very similar to L-arginine and is also present in red meats, chicken, and fish, but it is also present in melons, especially watermelon and highest in watermelon seed. L-cirtulline is converted in the body to L-arginine, which increases the production of NO. When L-arginine is combined with L-citrulline, NO output is actually increased. There is an L-citrulline/L-arginine recycling pathway that boosts NO production beyond when taking either L-arginine or L-citrulline alone. This is the reason I recommend that these two amino acids be taken together. The typical dose of L-cirtulline to lower blood pressure is 200 to 1,000 milligrams a day, but remember it works much better if combined with L-arginine. Watermelon seed is very rich in L-citrulline. (See Appendix C.)

Olive leaf extract

Traditionally olive leaf extract has been used as an antibiotic, antifungal, and antiviral treatment. Olive leaf supplements have been recommended for everything from nasal congestion to bowel problems. The active ingredient in olive leaf is oleuropein.[2]

Oleuropein has been shown to modulate the core cause of high blood pressure: arterial resistance or stiffness. One study showed that people with hypertension could experience reduced systolic blood pressure by an average 11.5 points mmHg, and diastolic blood pressure by 4.8 points—in just eight weeks—by taking olive leaf extract, in a dose of 500 milligrams twice a day.[3]

Flower extracts

- Hibiscus—People with high blood pressure (hypertension) can lower their blood pressure by drinking a tea made from a standardized extract of hibiscus flower every day, according to a study published in *Phytomedicine.*

  Hibiscus flowers have a fruity taste that makes hibiscus popular as both hot and cold tea. Studies have demonstrated that they have a diuretic property and have also found mild blood vessel-dilating effects. Several trials using hibiscus extracts have suggested that hibiscus can lower blood pressure in people with hypertension.

The current study evaluated seventy people with mild to moderate hypertension. Participants were randomly assigned to drink one-half liter (approximately 16 ounces) of hibiscus tea before breakfast each day or to take 25 milligrams of an antihypertensive medication (captopril) twice a day for four weeks. After four weeks the effectiveness of the two treatments was statistically similar: diastolic blood pressure (the lower number of a blood pressure reading) was reduced by at least ten points in 79 percent of the people receiving hibiscus and 84 percent of those receiving captopril.

The results of this study demonstrate that a tea made from a standardized hibiscus flower extract can reduce blood pressure in people with mild to moderate hypertension. Hibiscus flowers might have several components and properties that contribute to its blood-pressure-lowering effect. The antioxidants in hibiscus could add to its cardiovascular benefits by protecting blood vessels and heart muscle from oxidative damage. Furthermore, its safety and low potential for causing negative side effects make hibiscus an attractive alternative to antihypertensive medications.[4]

- Chrysanthemum—Chrysanthemum is a well-known medicinal herb in China. Clinical research conducted on the herb and its properties shows that the chrysanthemum is a very helpful remedy for the treatment of high blood pressure problems in patients. The Chinese have utilized herbal remedies made from the chrysanthemum for thousands of years. The chrysanthemum plant is indigenous to China and other Far Eastern countries—it grows in the wild in eastern Asia.

Chrysanthemum was extensively investigated in a number of Japanese- and Chinese-led clinical trials during the 1970s. These tests demonstrated that the chrysanthemum was quite effective in reducing elevated blood pressure.

Chrysanthemum contains alkaloids, volatile oil, sesquiterpene lactones, flavonoids, adenine, choline, stachydrine, chrysanthemin, and vitamin B_1.

The herbal infusion made from the chrysanthemum may be drunk thrice daily at a dosage of 200 milliliters or 8 ounces per dose. Dosages of this infusion recommended in Chinese medicine is about 4.5–15 grams or ¼–¾ ounces per dose per person on a daily basis.[5]

Beetroot juice

Drinking just 1 cup (or 8 ounces) of beetroot juice can help lower your blood pressure. The magic ingredient responsible for the impact on blood pressure is nitrate. Beetroots naturally contain high levels of it. Nitrate increases the levels nitric oxide in the bloodstream and is said to relax and widen the blood vessels and thereby improve blood pressure.[6] (See Appendix A.)

Other supplements that may help lower blood pressure include the extract of the Bonito fish (the peptides in this supplement work similarly to ACE inhibitor drugs but without the side effects[7]) and the C-12 peptide, which is a hydrolyzed or split milk protein. "Studies show that the C-12 peptide is a natural ACE inhibitor that has special blood pressure lowering effects.... But don't drink milk.

Instead take the C-12 peptide supplements that provides 200–400 mg/day."[8]

CRITICAL MINERALS

For over twenty years Americans with hypertension have been warned to limit sodium in their diets. Numerous studies have confirmed that a low-sodium diet lowers blood pressure if you are "sodium sensitive."[9]

Sodium controls the amount of fluid outside the cells and regulates the body's water balance and blood volume. Your kidneys actually regulate the amount of sodium in your body. When your sodium level is low, your kidneys begin to conserve sodium. When levels become high, your kidneys excrete the excess sodium in the urine.

Salt is the most common source of sodium. It is made up of approximately 60 percent chloride and 40 percent sodium. Your body requires about 500 milligrams of sodium every day, which is approximately a quarter of a teaspoon of salt. But Americans consume between 3,000 and 4,000 milligrams a day and on average 3,400 milligrams a day.

Too much sodium causes the body to retain water, so your blood volume increases similar to my prior analogy of opening up the faucet to increase the flow of water. The increased volume of blood then forces the heart to work harder, leading to increased resistance in the arteries, which in turn leads to high blood pressure. Limiting sodium intake to 2,300 milligrams or less a day or for some 1,500 milligrams a day will lower one's blood pressure 11.4/5.7 mmHg— that is pretty significant and lowers blood pressure as much as most blood pressure medications but without any side effects.

A **BIBLE CURE** *Health Fact*
Melatonin Lowers Blood Pressure

According to a study published by *Hypertension*, repeated oral intake of 2½ milligrams of melatonin one hour before sleep appears to lowers systolic and diastolic blood pressure by 4 to 6 mmHg. Melatonin plays a role in regulating your internal clock, which appears to be disturbed in people with high blood pressure.[10]

THE POWER OF POTASSIUM

Potassium is another mineral that helps to lower blood pressure. It also helps to keep your body's sodium level down to acceptable levels. That's why eating foods high in potassium, such as fresh fruits and vegetables, can help protect against high blood pressure.

Look for these high-potassium foods when you grocery shop:

- Beans (especially lima beans and soybeans)
- Tomatoes
- Prunes
- Avocados
- Bananas
- Peaches
- Cantaloupes

Also, a form of seaweed called dulse is extremely high in potassium. More than 4,000 milligrams of potassium are found in one-sixth of a cup! You can find dulse at your favorite health food store.

MAGNIFICENT MAGNESIUM

Magnesium is vital for healthy blood pressure and a robust cardio-vascular system. This powerful mineral is linked to more than 325 different enzyme reactions in the body. If your body is deficient in magnesium, you could be predisposed to developing hypertension, arrhythmias, and other cardiovascular conditions. Magnificent magnesium actually dilates arteries, thus decreasing blood pressure.

Are you magnesium deficient?

Many Americans are woefully lacking in magnesium. As a matter of fact, it is one of the most common deficiencies in the country, especially for the elderly.

Why? We drink too much coffee and alcohol, and we eat too many processed foods, all of which rob our bodies of this important mineral. For this reason I strongly recommend taking a magnesium supplement.

Take 400 milligrams of a chelated form such as magnesium glyci-nate, magnesium citrate, or magnesium aspartate once or twice a day.

Common sources of magnesium include nuts and seeds, green leafy vegetables, legumes, and whole grains. Let me caution you, however, that too much magnesium may cause diarrhea.

INCREDIBLE CALCIUM

Did you know that the most abundant mineral in your body is calcium? Calcium is critically important for maintaining the balance between your sodium and potassium and for regulating your blood pressure.

You can increase the amount of calcium in your diet by eating the following calcium-rich foods:

- Almonds
- Skim milk
- Skim milk cheeses
- Low-fat yogurt
- Sunflower seeds
- Soy
- Parsley
- Low-fat cottage cheese

Or try taking a daily calcium magnesium supplement containing 400 milligrams of calcium and 200 milligrams of magnesium two times a day. New studies are finding that consuming over 1,000 milligrams of calcium a day in foods and supplements can increase the risk of heart attack and stroke. So don't overdo it on calcium supplements, and don't consume excessive dairy products.

> Do not cast me off in the time of old age; do not forsake me when my strength fails.
>
> —PSALM 71:9

THE WONDERS OF WATER

Believe it or not, one of the best nutrients you can take for controlling your blood pressure is water.

When your body is lacking water, the water volume in every cell will be reduced, which then affects how efficiently nutrients and waste products are transported. What happens in the end is that our cells don't get enough nutrients, and they end up having too much waste collecting in them.

In addition, when you don't have enough water, your kidneys reabsorb more sodium. After you do drink fluids, this sodium in turn attracts and holds even more water, making the blood volume increase, which in turn may increase your blood pressure. It is similar to turning up the faucet to increase the flow of water.

If you don't drink enough water for too long, your body will begin to make certain adjustments to keep adequate blood flowing to your brain, heart, kidneys, liver, and lungs. Blood will be shunted away from less essential tissues and sent to the vital organs. Your body will actually divert water by constricting small arteries that lead to less essential tissues. In other words, your body will begin a water rationing program to make sure that enough blood goes to the vital organs first.

> God is the strength of my heart and my portion forever.
>
> —PSALM 73:26

Think of it like this: when you constrict a water hose by bending it or by pressing your thumb over the opening, what happens? The pressure behind that constriction increases dramatically, doesn't it? Your arteries behave in a similar way. Therefore, increasing your intake of water helps to open up your smaller arteries and helps to prevent this rise in blood pressure.

Often an individual with mild hypertension is placed on medication when all he really needs is to drink more water. When high blood pressure is detected early enough, simply drinking 2 to 3 quarts of alkaline water a day can usually bring it back to normal.

What's even worse than medicating a person who just needs water is placing such an individual on diuretics, which happens all the time.

They lose even more water as well as valuable electrolytes including potassium and magnesium.

Eight glasses of water a day to help keep high blood pressure away

If you have high blood pressure, drink at least eight to twelve glasses of alkaline water a day. The best time to drink water is thirty minutes before meals and two hours after meals. However, if you have kidney disease or a weak heart, you will need to limit your water intake, and you should be under the care of a physician.

HYPERTENSION MEDICATIONS

The best way to control your blood pressure is through changes in diet and lifestyle, lowering your salt intake, increasing your water intake, taking the nutritional supplements to lower blood pressure, reducing stress, and decreasing your weight, especially belly fat. But if after doing all the above you find that your blood pressure is still elevated, you may need the help of medication. Realize, however, that all hypertensive medications may have side effects. Approximately 68 million Americans have hypertension, but only about 47 percent of them have it controlled with medication. It's critically important to work with your doctor and find a medicine that's right for you.

In addition, if you have high blood pressure, I strongly recommend that you visit a nutritional doctor—either a nutritional medical doctor, a doctor of osteopathy, or a naturopath—who can use stress reduction, weight control, nutritional therapy, aerobic exercise, and adequate water intake as a first line of therapy for controlling hypertension.

CONCLUSION

Supplements, nutrients, water, stress reduction, diet and lifestyle changes, and weight reduction can powerfully strengthen your body against the ravages of high blood pressure. But your greatest source of strength is God Himself. The Bible says that those who look to Him for strength will not be disappointed. "Blessed is the man whose strength is in You, whose heart is set on pilgrimage.... They go from strength to strength" (Ps. 84:5, 7).

Would you like to feel as if you go from strength to strength, blasting through every obstacle you encounter with God's power and might? If so, always look to God for your strength, wisdom, power, and understanding. As the Creator of your very unique body He will lead you to supplements, nutrients, and everything else your body needs to lower your blood pressure and live strong past the threescore and ten years that we are all promised.

A **BIBLE CURE** Prayer for You

Dear God, I thank You that You've created me to be the object of Your great love and affection. Be my strength every day of my life, and let me live to go from strength to strength. Thank You for being a shield and protector for my life and health. Thank You for providing strength and help for my body. I pray for the power of discipline to be faithful to all of the wisdom You are teaching me through this book. Amen.

A **BIBLE CURE** *Prescription*

Describe the changes you plan to make after reading this chapter.

_____

_____

_____

The Bible says that God is your protector and your shield. How does that apply personally to your own situation of high blood pressure?

_____

_____

_____

Do you believe that God is a healer? Why?

_____

_____

_____

Chapter 5

YOUR HEART AND STRESS

ANY YEARS AGO my pastor would sometimes ask me to address the church on health topics. By the time I walked onto the platform I would be drenched in sweat, feeling as if I wanted to run out the nearest exit door and disappear into the night so I wouldn't have to face the few hundred people in the audience. I was terrified of public speaking. I remember my pastor putting his hand on my shoulder one time and saying, "You're perspiring terribly. Is it that hot in here?" I didn't have the guts to tell him I was scared to death to be under the spotlight with him. Those moments of stress and plenty of other hard-earned stress lessons from my own life have taught me a lot about the subject.

Some people go through life stressed. Just driving in heavy traffic stresses them out; so does saying hello to a neighbor or calling to inquire about a bill. That stress reaction, so useful in moments of actual emergency, becomes a self-destruct switch that eventually can lead to exhaustion and disease, such as high blood pressure.

GOOD STRESS AND BAD STRESS

There are two types of stress—*eustress* and *distress*.[1] Eustress is good stress, such as falling in love, that motivates and inspires. Distress is bad stress and can be short-lived or chronic. Dr. Hans Selye observed that if a situation is perceived as very good or very bad, then demands are placed upon the mind and the body accordingly to adapt to the situation.

Stress is also our body's natural reaction to a threat or perceived threat. It causes a sudden release of adrenaline and other hormones that cause your blood pressure to go up, your heart to beat faster, and your lungs to take in more air among other physiologic events. These stress hormones give you extra strength and mental acuity for a few moments, and they empower you to either fight or flee.

But when the stress response occurs too frequently or goes on long term, those stress hormones that were meant to save your life begin to actually harm you. They can leave you feeling depressed, anxious, angry, with low sex drive, and predisposed to obesity, type 2 diabetes, high cholesterol, hypertension, and all kinds of illnesses. The same hormones that save your life in an emergency can actually begin to destroy your health if the stress response does not turn off. Many people are triggering this stress response repeatedly for minor, insignificant problems or by feeling frustrated, irritated, angry, anxious, fearful, resentful, or bitter. They are burning ten dollars worth of hormonal rocket fuel (figuratively speaking) for a two-cent problem. It is also raising their blood pressure by chronically stimulating their stress response. We are designed for this stress response to happen during true emergencies and not for minor problems or toxic emotions.

CONSEQUENCES OF STRESS

In June 2005 the *Wall Street Journal* devoted an entire section of their newspaper to how to live longer. The front-page article of the section said, "Increasingly, researchers are viewing stress—how much stress we face in a lifetime, and how well we cope with it—as one of the most significant factors for predicting how well we age."[2] The article concluded that stress "kills" people as much or more than poor health habits such as smoking, drinking alcohol, or not exercising.

Stress is not just a mental problem; it's the cause of many of the diseases and maladies I treat in my practice. Many recent studies have demonstrated this. The renowned Nun Study has shown that elevated stress levels inhibit and deteriorate the hippocampus, the part of the brain associated with memory and learning. A smaller hippocampus is a sign of Alzheimer's disease.[3]

A long-term study at the University of London showed that chronic unmanaged mental stress was six times more predictive of cancer and heart disease than cigarette smoking, high cholesterol levels, and elevated blood pressure.[4] In a Mayo Clinic study of people with heart disease, psychological stress was the strongest predictor of future cardiac events.[5] In a ten-year study people who were not able to manage their stress effectively had a 40 percent higher death rate than those who were "unstressed."[6]

Stress, strokes, and sickness

Excessive stress long term can make you obese and unhealthy. In response to long-term stress the hormone cortisol rises, which can cause the blood pressure to rise, can cause the release of fats and sugar in the bloodstream, and may cause weight gain, elevated triglycerides, high cholesterol, and elevated blood sugar. Cortisol may save your life if you are a POW or experiencing famine, because it slows your metabolic rate and helps to preserve your fat stores. But most of us aren't POWs or experiencing famine, and so the high cortisol levels usually lead to weight gain especially in the belly.

Stressed-out people also tend to develop brown marks under their eyes and frown lines on their foreheads, around the eyes, and around the mouth. Some even get bulging eyes, a tight jaw, and flared nostrils. Plastic surgeons are cashing in on the stress epidemic, performing facelifts and offering Botox injections and more.

> Be anxious for nothing, but in everything by prayer and supplication, with thanksgiving, let your requests be made known to God.
>
> —PHILIPPIANS 4:6

Cortisol affects the "control loop" that regulates the sex hormones. Elevated cortisol is associated with a drop in DHEA and testosterone, which can lead to a decreased sex drive and erectile dysfunction. In women elevated cortisol is associated with lower levels of progesterone and testosterone. During periods of chronic stress, progesterone is actually converted to cortisol in the body, which can lead to a progesterone deficiency. This, in turn, can lead to menstrual problems and PMS, as well as significant menopausal symptoms such as hot flashes and night sweats. Levels of estrogen become imbalanced in the presence of high cortisol.

Chronic stress also has commonly been associated with depression. Elevated cortisol levels cause an imbalance of neurotransmitters in the brain, notably serotonin and dopamine. In one scientific study as many as seven out of every ten patients with depression had enlarged adrenal glands, some with glands that were 1.7 times the size of a normal gland in a person who is not depressed.[7] In other words, the adrenal gland had enlarged in response to the demand for more cortisol. The cortisol, in turn, causes an imbalance of these important neurotransmitters.

Excessive stress can predispose a person to develop or aggravate every conceivable affliction. Clearly, disease and illness are often the shrapnel wounds from stress. If you want to manage your stress, you must first learn to identify causes of stress.

Causes of stress

The causes of stress are all too familiar to most Americans. Trouble with finances, relationships, job problems, health, or sudden traumatic events head the list, followed by a myriad of minor stressors such as computer trouble, traffic, poor customer service, dirty laundry stacking up, cleaning house, driving children to extracurricular activities, ongoing conflict with friends or family members, loneliness, or even aggravating lights or noise near your home.

WHAT STRESS LOOKS LIKE ON YOU

Dr. Selye experimented with rats using different physical stressors such as electrical shocks and cold temperature. By doing this he discovered that if stress was maintained long enough, the body would go through three stages. These stages include the alarm stage, the resistance stage, and the exhaustion stage.

STAGE ONE: ALARM

In the early 1900s Dr. Walter Cannon of Harvard University first coined the phrase "fight-or-flight response." This is now known as the stress response, which is a kind of intricate and elaborate emergency alarm system that God created in your body. It is actually a survival response placed in us by God for our protection.

The fight-or-flight response actually begins in the hypothalamus, which is an area of the brain involved in survival. When you encounter a dangerous situation, such as being attacked by a bear, your hypothalamus signals your pituitary gland to secrete a hormone that in turn activates the adrenal glands. These glands release adrenaline, which is epinephrine. I'm sure you've heard someone say that he was operating on adrenaline. This is what that person was referring to.

This fight-or-flight response signals massive changes. Your entire body goes on high alert.

- Your muscles tighten and get tense.
- Your heart rate increases.
- Your blood vessels constrict.
- Your blood pressure rises.
- Breathing becomes faster and deeper.
- Perspiration increases.
- Blood is shunted away from the stomach so that digestion is slowed or halted.
- Blood sugar and fat are dumped into the bloodstream for extra energy.
- Fats rise in the blood.
- The thyroid gland is stimulated.
- The secretion of saliva is slowed down.
- The brain becomes more alert.
- Sensory perception becomes sharper.
- Blood is shunted to the muscles and away from the digestive tract so digestion slows or stops.
- The colon increases peristalsis so that you can dump your load to run faster.

This alarm reaction can save your life. If you see a rattlesnake while hiking, you are able to run to safety. If you're camping and get attacked by a bear, you can get away and survive. This incredible alarm system may allow you to escape from disaster by secreting these powerful hormones that provide tremendous strength and energy.

We have all heard the accounts of the grandmother who lifted a car off of her elderly husband after the jack slipped and the car pinned him underneath. Fantastic though they sound, these stories are true. They reveal the power of this incredible stress system to respond to danger.

I actually had one patient who was carjacked. As she was being driven to a remote area, she jumped out of the car as it was moving and was able to run to safety. This survival response that God placed in us for our protection works in similar fashion to the passing gear in a car. It empowers us with a burst of near superhuman power and strength in order to overcome adversity by fighting or fleeing. However, if you are stressing over minor circumstances or are frustrated, irritated, angry, anxious, fearful, or bitter, the alarm reaction is occurring many times a day and raising your blood pressure each time. This can eventually lead to hypertension.

STAGE TWO: RESISTANCE

If the body's alarm response becomes more and more frequent, it leads to the second stage of stress, which is known as the resistance stage. This, again, is a natural survival response placed in us by God to help us survive without adequate nutrition, as during times of famine, war, and pestilence.

In 2 Kings 25:1–4 we read about a siege upon the Jews by Babylon that lasted for one and a half years. During this time the people lacked food. These ancient citizens of Jerusalem experienced this stage two survival response. This response begins when an individual perceives that he or she has lost control. In modern life it's seen when a person encounters considerable financial stress with no way out, seriously failing health, the loss of a job, divorce or separation, a sick child or wife, a child in rebellion, or some other traumatic event where an individual perceives a long-term loss of control.

Gearing up to survive

Remember that this second stage is a survival mechanism that we are programmed with to survive some long-term crisis such as a war, famine, or drought. The hormone cortisol is released constantly to enable you to cope with chronic, unremitting stress.

So what happens at this stage?

- Your hypothalamus is stimulated.
- This in turn stimulates the pituitary gland.
- A prolonged increase of both the hormones cortisol and adrenaline are released, but mainly cortisol.
- The cortisol actually causes a decreased sensitivity of the brain centers for feedback inhibition (so the stress response doesn't turn off and more cortisol is produced).
- This leads to prolonged elevation of cortisol.
- Blood sugar is usually elevated.

As your blood sugar level is increased over time, insulin resistance can occur, leading to type 2 diabetes. It also leads to increased bone loss, an elevation in blood fats such as triglycerides and cholesterol, and an increased accumulation of fat, especially around the waist, leading to "apple-shaped obesity."

The resistance stage also leads to an increased breakdown of proteins that can cause muscle wasting, especially in the arms, legs, and other large muscle groups. At this point your immune system can begin to falter and fail as the levels of immune cells become increasingly depleted.

During the resistance stage the prolonged increase of adrenaline and cortisol leads to a loss of magnesium, potassium, and calcium and to sodium retention. These minerals are extremely important for blood pressure control. Without them blood pressure usually remains elevated. Sodium retention also raises the blood pressure. As the levels of both cortisol and adrenaline remain high, eventually hypertension and heart disease can result.

STAGE THREE: EXHAUSTION

As the body activates the sympathetic nervous system over such a long period of time without giving it a break, eventually the adrenal glands become depleted. The two powerful hormones that started and sustained this process for so long now begin to become depleted. Both cortisol and adrenaline levels decline.

When your body cannot go anymore

Your body has launched and sustained all of its resources for a very long time. Now it simply begins to wear out—and sometimes it can wear out rather quickly. Think about it in this way: imagine getting into your car and pressing the gas pedal to the floor for hours while the car is in park with its engine running. No doubt it would take quite a toll on the engine. Now think about what would happen to the engine if you sustained this for days or weeks. It wouldn't be long before the engine began to break down in significant ways, and it certainly wouldn't be long before the car was out of gas. People stuck in this exhaustion stage are similar to a car with its accelerator pressed to the floor, and now it's out of gas.

When your body is forced to deal with the biochemical storm created by stress for a sustained period of time, the same thing occurs—your once robust, powerful body that was designed to last for many, many years begins to break down prematurely.

If you are a stressed-out person in stage three exhaustion, here's what you might expect. You may begin to experience hypoglycemia, which is low blood sugar. In addition, poor fat and protein absorption in your body could lead to the loss of muscle mass.

With time your immune system will become depleted, and you may experience some of the following symptoms:

- Allergies to foods, inhalants, and chemicals
- Inflammation, joint aches and pains, rashes, muscle aches
- Lower resistance to infection and recurrent infections such as recurrent colds, sinus infections, and viral infections, including chronic mono and yeast infections
- Severe fatigue
- Anxiety
- Irritability
- Memory problems
- Problems sleeping
- Digestive problems—bloating, gas, diarrhea, constipation

During this stage you can be very susceptible to infections (bacterial and viral infections such as chronic sinusitis, recurrent bronchitis, and pharyngitis), allergies (environmental and food), autoimmune diseases (such as rheumatoid arthritis, lupus, thyroid-itis, and multiple sclerosis) and cancer. Organ systems may also begin to fail during this stage. During this stage, inflammation is usually rampant in the body since not enough cortisol is present to quench the inflammation. Excessive inflammation may lead to hypertension and heart disease as well as chronic pain, which also usually raises the blood pressure even more. For more information on how to overcome stress, please refer to my books *Stress Less* and *The New Bible Cure for Stress*.

CONCLUSION

While this may seem like a lot of information to take in, having an understanding about how your body responds during challenging situations—whether actual or perceived—is critical in your making the necessary adjustments to the way you respond mentally and emotionally. It is wonderful to know that God knows us. He knows us inside and out and has provided us with a road map to the place of peace in His Son, Jesus Christ. Now let's move on to discovering how we can combat the effects of modern stress.

A BIBLE CURE Prayer for You

Dear God, thank You so much that You are providing me with knowledge on how stress affects my body. Now, because You are my Creator, I ask that You lead me to the way of peace and contentment. I ask that You help me learn how to cast all my cares on You, because You care for me. I thank You in advance for Your peace that passes all understanding that will guard my heart and mind. In Jesus's name I pray, amen.

A **BIBLE CURE** *Prescription*

Take a moment and list the things that are currently causing you stress, things you may be worried about. Now according to Philippians 4:6–7: "Be anxious for nothing...and the peace of God, which surpasses all understanding, will guard your hearts and minds through Christ Jesus."

_____

_____

_____

_____

_____

_____

_____

Chapter 6

COMBAT MODERN STRESS
AT THE ROOT

Since today's stress generally has a large psychological and emotional component, getting it under control so that it cannot overdrive the body's organ systems requires hitting it at the roots.

Long-term stress is rooted in the perception that you've lost control. Therefore, to manage stress it is critical that you develop a perception of control over your life. Studies have found that individuals with excessive stress on the job have more hypertension.[1] But it's not really the stress. Two people can encounter the same circumstances, and one may be overwhelmed with stress while the other one remains completely undisturbed. It's not actually stress of the work, but the perception of loss of control that causes blood pressure to rise. Here are several ways to adjust your perceptions, correct wrong thinking, and live in peace.

ACTIVATE THE POWER OF GOD'S WORD

Since stress is rooted in the perception of loss of control, renewing your mind with the Word of God will yank up stress by the roots. In other words, stress begins in the mind, and the Word of God has the power to shield, protect, and strengthen the mind against the power of stress.

The Bible contains living words of truth and power spoken by a living God who loves you and longs to see you walk in wholeness and health. When you feel stressed out, look up and read Galatians 5:16–26 to help you take control of your thoughts.

CONTROL EVERY THOUGHT

The Bible promises us that we can control every anxious, worried, fretful, and fearful thought. We don't have to let stress get the upper hand in our minds.

Here are two powerful scriptures to read aloud when stress begins to assault your thoughts:

> Casting down arguments and every high thing that exalts itself against the knowledge of God, bringing every thought into captivity to the obedience of Christ.
>
> —2 CORINTHIANS 10:5

> Finally, brethren, whatever things are true, whatever things are noble, whatever things are just, whatever things are pure, whatever things are lovely, whatever things are of good report, if there is any virtue and if there is anything praiseworthy—meditate on these things.
>
> —PHILIPPIANS 4:8

Let Jesus be the gatekeeper of your mind. Unless a thought passes all the criteria listed above, only then should it be allowed entrance into the mind to be meditated on and rehashed.

In Your presence is fullness of joy.

—PSALM 16:11

LIVE IN THE PRESENT

Many times stress comes from worry about tomorrow. Jesus said in Matthew 6:34: "Do not worry about tomorrow, for tomorrow will worry about its own things. Sufficient for the day is its own trouble." Not taking the Lord's advice on this has led a lot of people into living a stress-filled life rather than the peace-filled life He died to give us. To help my patients combat worrying, I encourage them to practice mindfulness—the practice of learning to pay attention to what is happening to you from moment to moment.

Mindfulness is a biblical practice. The apostle Paul taught us to forget "those things which are behind" (Phil. 3:13), meaning the past. Mindfulness means letting go of any thought that is unrelated to the present moment and finding something to enjoy in the present moment.

Unfortunately most people do not live in the present moment. They are thinking such things as: "I'll be happy when..."

- "I get a bigger place to live."
- "I get that promotion."
- "My kids are out of school."
- "I pay off these bills."
- "I get a new car."

Mindfulness helps you to stop complaining about what you don't have and to start practicing gratitude for what you do have.

As you practice mindfulness, your muscles will relax, your body unwinds, and your stress is relieved. Make mindfulness a habit by practicing it daily.

TAME YOUR TONGUE

In addition to taking control of your mind, you must also begin to tame your tongue and quit letting your words be the vehicles upon which stressful thoughts travel.

Here are some powerful verses for you to memorize:

Out of the abundance of the heart the mouth speaks.

—Matthew 12:34

Every idle word men may speak, they shall give account of it in the day of judgment.

—Matthew 12:36

Let no corrupt word proceed out of your mouth.

—Ephesians 4:29

Death and life are in the power of the tongue.

—Proverbs 18:21

BE QUICK TO FORGIVE

One of the secret causes of stress plaguing millions of people is unforgiveness. People rehash the wrong that was done to them, or that they misperceive was done to them, and their bodies immediately have stress responses. When you fail to forgive, you lock yourself into long-term stress response similar to pulling a scab off a sore so that it never heals. Your body is literally stewing in its own stress juices every time you relive a wrong that was done to you.

The apostle Paul wrote, "Bearing with one another, and forgiving one another, if anyone has a complaint against another; even as Christ forgave you, so you also must do" (Col. 3:13). To forgive does not mean that you didn't get hurt. Rather, it's choosing not to live in the feeling of unforgiveness. You can trust God to deal with the offense and the offender. If you continue to hold on to unforgiveness toward someone else, you do not hurt that other person; you damage your own health and invite hypertension and heart disease into your body. Therefore, you should release your anger and bitterness for the sake of self-preservation. I strongly recommend my books *Deadly Emotions* and *Stress Less*.

GET A FRESH PERSPECTIVE

Another way to handle the stress is by reframing, which is all about learning to see the past, present, and future in a positive light. Reframing calls upon a person to shift his focus away from his present point of view in order to "see" something from a new perspective.

James, the brother of Jesus, taught us the meaning of reframing when we face trials:

> My brethren, count it all joy when you fall into various trials, knowing that the testing of your faith produces patience.
>
> —JAMES 1:2–3

James was giving us God's perspective. Scriptural reframing is one of the most powerful ways to relieve stress. It is simply replacing our fears, worries, failures, grief, sorrows, and shame with God's promises.

Reframing your thoughts can have a very real effect on your heart. The heart is much more than a pump; it also functions as a hormonal gland, a sensory organ, and an information-encoding and -processing center.

When you experience stress and negative emotions such as anger, frustration, fear, and anxiety, your heart rate variability pattern becomes more erratic and disordered, and it sends chaotic signals to the brain. This causes your system to get "out of sync." The result is excessive stress with toxic emotions, energy drain, and added wear and tear on your mind and body. In contrast, sustained positive emotions, such as appreciation, love, joy, and compassion, are associated with highly ordered patterns on the heart rate variability tracing and a significant reduction of stress.

According to the Institute of HeartMath, these core heart feelings of gratitude, joy, peace, and love increase synchronization and coherence in the heart rhythm patterns, and these in turn decrease stress and will help to lower one's blood pressure. For more on this topic of HeartMath see my book *Stress Less*.

BE A GOOD STEWARD OF YOUR TIME

Time is ultimately your most precious possession. Many people stay stressed because they fail to organize their time. This is so simple to do, but some people don't know where to begin. I recommend these steps:

1. Purchase a calendar "organizer" or put that smartphone or tablet to good use to keep track of key dates such as birthdays and anniversaries, as well as deadlines and dates of major events.

2. Organize your desk at work and home. The average office worker spends three hours a week sorting piles trying to locate which project to work on next![2]

3. Throw away junk mail daily.

4. Buy a filing cabinet or organizing system for storing important papers, articles, warranties, documents, deeds, wills, and other valuable items.

5. Organize your kitchen, and meal preparation will be easier and faster.

6. Turn off your phone during certain hours to avoid taking calls that are a total waste of your time.

7. Declare one day a week, or perhaps one weekend a month, as a media "fast" time—no computer, no television, no radio, no news, and no videos or DVDs. Use this time to connect with your family or friends.

8. Make the most of your "waiting" times. It may be a doctor's office or a dentist's office, an appointment at the bank, or at the airport. Always have a book, magazine, tape, or piece of handwork available to fill this time with something positive and productive.

9. Limit the amount of time you spend with negative, pessimistic people. They not only will sabotage your goals, but they will also drain energy from you.

10. Refuse to be distracted if you are focused on a work project. Turn your phone off. Close your door. Don't allow for interruptions. You get more done in an hour of totally focused time without interruptions than in three hours of time that has only a few interruptions.

11. Make a to-do list each evening before you go to bed. This way you don't need to continue to mull things over in your mind all night.

12. Make dining an experience by tasting, smelling, and savoring every bite of food instead of wolfing it down. Avoid arguments and stressful topics at mealtime. Avoid eating on the run or as you drive your car. A great deal of stress can be eliminated if a person will simply use mealtimes as opportunities to relax, daydream a little, and rest.

WALK IN THE POWER OF LOVE

One of the greatest powers available to you is the power of love. Love can free you of fear, which stress is often rooted in.

> There is no fear in love; but perfect love casts out fear.
> —1 JOHN 4:18

Do you feel alone and needing love? We all need love. You may find that one wonderful way to surround your life with love is to own a loving pet. When you get home from work, it will always be there waiting, eager to see you and always by your side. You may find that holding your adoring animal on your lap causes the stress of your hectic day to melt away.

You can't be selfish when you love, for love has to be given away. And one of the best ways to lower your stress is to give and receive love. Make every effort to give away God's pure love. Hug your spouse or a friend, hold hands with your child, give an elderly person a loving touch. Express the love of Christ often, and ask God for opportunities to give His love away.

HAVE A GOOD LAUGH

Laughter releases chemicals in the brain that can help to relieve pain and create a sense of well-being. Laughter also strengthens the heart, lungs and muscles. In fact, Norman Cousins referred to laughter as internal jogging.[3] Just twenty seconds of laughter produces an exchange of oxygen equal to about twenty minutes of aerobic exercise.

I believe laughter is the best medicine for relieving stress and hypertension. One of the most unusual prescriptions I give to many of my patients is to have at least ten belly laughs a day.

True laughing offers one of the most powerful and natural healing methods without any side effects. Laughter lowers the stress hormones cortisol and epinephrine (adrenaline) and increases feel-good hormones (endorphins). These are the same hormones runners seek and are called the runner's high.

Laughter keeps you squarely in the present moment. It helps you to reframe and feel thankful and helps you to see negative events in a more positive light. There's not a single bad thing laughter will do for your body and mind.

The Bible declares:

> Rejoice in the Lord always. Again I will say, rejoice!
> —PHILIPPIANS 4:4

> The joy of the LORD is your strength!
> —NEHEMIAH 8:10

A good hearty laugh can help:

- Reduce stress
- Lower blood pressure
- Elevate mood
- Boost the immune system
- Improve brain functioning
- Protect the heart
- Connect you to others
- Foster instant relaxation
- Make you feel good[4]

If you are stressed out or depressed, or if you have high blood pressure, learn to laugh. Go to funny movies, watch funny, clean TV shows, tell jokes, get joke books, and read comic sections in the newspaper. Laughter is truly the best medicine for overcoming stress and helping to lower your blood pressure.

CONCLUSION

In this chapter you have sees that stress is manageable. Laughing is one of the best remedies for a heavy heart. Follow the tips in this chapter that give you the best results, and develop a pattern to always take matters to God in prayer. He is your help and your guide. With Him in your heart, you are never alone.

A **BIBLE CURE** Prayer for You

Dear Lord, You know my thoughts and my heart. You know my rising up and my lying down. Lord, I ask that You help me navigate my way to a stress-free life in You. I know this is part of Your perfect plan for me. Help me to discern the best way for me to lead a peaceful and happy life. Thank you so much for providing me with a way out of the modern stress cycle that plagues so many. Amen.

A **BIBLE CURE** *Prescription*
7 Tips to Beginning a Stress-Less Life

1. Identify what things you can control and what things are beyond your control.

2. Compile a list of ten things for which you are grateful. Then post the list where you can see it throughout the day (like on your bathroom mirror or on the refrigerator door).

3. Instead of seeing disappointments, setbacks, and trials as a time to complain, worry, or criticize, begin to reframe and see these events as teachers. What did this situation teach you so that you can avoid that mistake next time around?

4. Find a TV show, DVD, or movie with clean humor, watch it tonight, and laugh a lot!

5. Whatever you need to accomplish today, allow for margin in your tasks. Make a "to-do" list; give yourself plenty of time to get from one destination to another. Prioritize your schedule and decide on what you can postpone for another day.

6. Take five minutes today to practice abdominal breathing. To learn how to do this, lie down on your back in a comfortable position and place your left hand on your abdomen and your right hand on your chest. First, practice filling your lower lungs by allowing your abdomen to push out your left hand, which causes your abdominal cavity to expand. Your right hand on your

chest should remain still. Make sure your breathing is slow and steady. About ten slow, deep abdominal breaths will leave you feeling relaxed and calm. I recommend that you practice this nightly for five to ten minutes, and eventually you will be able to do it when stressed while sitting, standing, or even talking. If you find yourself in a stressful situation, take a moment to practice some deep breathing before you react.

7. Today is your day of jubilee, so thank Him aloud for His goodness! By continuing to practice biblical principles, you will begin to walk in divine health.

Chapter 7

ACTIVATE THE POWER OF DYNAMIC FAITH OVER YOUR HEALTH

'D LIKE TO share with you one of the most powerful scriptures in the Bible. It says, "The eyes of the LORD run to and fro throughout the whole earth, to show Himself strong on behalf of those whose heart is loyal to Him" (2 Chron. 16:9).

What this means is this: when you commit your heart to God, He is always looking for ways to make you stronger—and He has the entire earth at His disposal. This is important because it means that you can trust God to strengthen your body and your life, even against a physical assault of high blood pressure.

God's eye is on the sparrow. The Bible says, "Are not five sparrows sold for two copper coins? And not one of them is forgotten before God. But the very hairs of your head are all numbered. Do not fear therefore; you are of more value than many sparrows" (Luke 12:6–7).

Not a tiny sparrow flies through the sky that God doesn't watch over. If He sees them and cares deeply for their every need, how much more does He watch over you? He cares for your every need—the needs of your body, your mind, and your spirit.

Having faith in God's unwavering love for you is the last Bible cure key to freedom from high blood pressure.

Many people believe faith is some eerie power that some have while others do not. That's simply not true. Faith is nothing more than a choice to believe God and take Him at His Word—the Bible. Faith in action makes the choice to believe God no matter what the circumstances say, no matter what your feelings and emotions say, no matter what your friends say. Faith looks beyond the natural realm and touches the supernatural when it chooses to believe. It's really so simple!

FAITH FOR ALL THAT CONCERNS YOU

Some people believe that they can have faith for salvation, but otherwise they feel that God has pretty much left them on their own. But if God cares deeply for a tiny sparrow, and if He has numbered all the hairs on your head, do you really think He doesn't care about your other health issues? Of course He does. He cares greatly about all of them—even your high blood pressure!

I believe that is why God has led me to write this and other Bible Cure books, because God truly does care very deeply about you and your health. He is a wonderful Creator who created your body to function well for you. He also wants you to have the necessary wisdom and understanding to keep it functioning well for a very long time. Good health—that's God's plan for you because He loves you. He even wishes above all things that you prosper and be in health, even as your soul prospers (3 John 2).

GOD'S LOVE AND YOUR HEALTH

Understanding God's love for you can have a powerful impact upon your health. When you truly begin to trust God for the many details of your life, you will begin to discover a peace in your life that has many powerful benefits to your soul, your mind and, yes, to your health. When you know how much God loves you, you will rest from the anxious striving and worry of life. Not only will you be happier, but you will also be much healthier.

High blood pressure is not a life sentence. I believe that you will overcome high blood pressure and go forward to develop a healthier lifestyle in many ways. Let's pray now and ask God to confirm this in your heart.

A **BIBLE CURE** Prayer for You

Dear Jesus, I thank You for the power of Your love and the peace of Your presence in my life. I pray that You will increase my faith to trust You with the details of my life. I surrender my cares and worries to You in exchange for Your joy and peace. Thank You, God, for paving a clear path for me to complete wholeness and healing. In Your name, amen.

A **BIBLE CURE** Prescription

Now that you have asked God to reveal His love and peace to you, make a list of the ways that He has shown His love for you through blessings, opportunities, good relationships, or special provision.

A Personal Note

FROM DON AND MARY COLBERT

G OD DESIRES TO heal you of disease. His Word is full of promises that confirm His love for you and His desire to give you His abundant life. His desire includes more than physical health for you; He wants to make you whole in your mind and spirit as well through a personal relationship with His Son, Jesus Christ.

If you haven't met my best friend, Jesus, I would like to take this opportunity to introduce Him to you. It is very simple. If you are ready to let Him come into your life and become your best friend, all you need to do is sincerely pray this prayer:

> *Lord Jesus, I want to know You as my Savior and Lord. I believe You are the Son of God and that You died for my sins. I also believe You were raised from the dead and now sit at the right hand of the Father praying for me. I ask You to forgive me for my sins and change my heart so that I can be Your child and live with You eternally. Thank You for Your peace. Help me to walk with You so that I can begin to know You as my best friend and my Lord. Amen.*

If you have prayed this prayer, you have just made the most important decision of your life. I rejoice with you in your decision and your new relationship with Jesus. Please contact my publisher at pray4me@charismamedia.com so that we can send you some materials that will help you become established in your relationship with the Lord. We look forward to hearing from you.

Appendix A

SUPERFOODS FOR YOUR HEART

WHAT YOU EAT is the single most important factor when it comes to your health. Here are a few stand-out foods that will help to lower your blood pressure and promote overall heart health.[1]

ORGANIC CELERY

Celery is an excellent source of antioxidant nutrients such as vitamin C, beta-carotene, and manganese. But what really makes it stand out as a heart-healthy food is its phytonutrients. Many of these phytonutrients fall into the category of phenolic antioxidants and have been shown to provide anti-inflammatory benefits as well.[2]

Celery is a traditional Asian folk remedy for high blood pressure. It's possible that celery may work only if your high blood pressure is caused by too much renin in your blood produced by your kidneys.

If your blood pressure is high because of elevated renin levels and you are given a diuretic for your initial treatment, this could make your blood pressure soar even higher. Find out first if the high blood pressure is caused by too much renin, then consider making celery a part of your high blood pressure treatment plan.

In the book *The New Healing Herbs* a story is told about Mr. Minh Le who ate four celery stalks for one week and took three weeks off to help lower his high blood pressure. Mr. Le saw his blood pressure drop from 158/96 to 118/82 within one week.

By way of his son, Mr. Minh Le brought this ancient Chinese remedy to researchers to test at the University of Chicago Medical Center. The investigators tested animals by injecting the mammals with a small amount of 3-n-butyl phthalide, a chemical compound that is found in celery. Mr. Minh Le's son, Quang Le, and University of Chicago pharmacologist William Elliot, PhD, isolated the compound 3-n-butyl phthalide and injected rats with the equivalent amount of what's found in four stalks of celery.

Not only did the rats' blood pressure drop 13 percent in a week, but the rats' cholesterol levels also dropped by 7 percent. The chemical that reduced the animals' blood pressure readings turned out to be phthalide. It's known in scientific circles that phthalide relaxes the muscles and arteries that regulate blood pressure. Phthalide is a chemical that also reduced the amount of "stress hormones," called catecholamines. Stress hormones also raise blood pressure since catecholamines constrict blood vessels.

One stalk of celery does contain about 35 milligrams of sodium, which should not raise your blood pressure. Be sure to choose organic celery since celery is typically high in pesticide residue.[3]

BEETROOT JUICE

Boosting stamina and energy, improving blood flood, and reducing blood pressure, beetroot juice is one of the richest dietary sources of antioxidants and nitrates that improve blood pressure and blood flow throughout the body, including the brain, heart, muscles, and more.[4]

Drinking just 1 cup (or 8 ounces) of beetroot juice can help lower your blood pressure. A study found that participants with high blood pressure experienced a decrease of about 10 mmHg following a daily dose of the juice. The magic ingredient responsible for the impact on blood pressure is nitrate. Beetroots naturally contain high levels of it. Nitrate increases the levels of nitric oxide in the bloodstream and is said to relax and widen the blood vessels and thereby improve blood pressure.[5]

GARLIC

Garlic is used for many conditions related to the heart and circulatory system, including high blood pressure, high cholesterol, coronary heart disease, heart attack, and "hardening of the arteries" (atherosclerosis). Studies have shown that garlic is effective in slowing the development of atherosclerosis and reducing blood pressure.

Not all garlic products sold for medicinal purposes are the same. In order for garlic to be effective in reversing heart conditions, it must have the right amount of allicin, which also happens to be the active ingredient that gives garlic its distinctive order. Odorless garlic supplements reduce the amount of allicin and compromise the effectiveness of the product. Methods that involve crushing the fresh clove release more allicin.[6]

EXTRA-VIRGIN OLIVE OIL

The monounsaturated fats in olive oil help lower your risk of heart disease by lowering total cholesterol and low-density lipoprotein cholesterol levels. It also helps with normalizing blood clotting.[7]

People on high blood pressure medications may be able to reduce the amount of medicine they take if they substitute extra-virgin olive oil for other types of fats in their diet. According to research, about 40 grams per day of extra-virgin olive oil markedly reduces the dosage of blood pressure medication by about 50 percent in hypertensive patients on a previously stable drug dosage. Forty grams per day of extra-virgin olive oil amount to about 4 tablespoons. Only extra-virgin olive oil contains antioxidants called "polyphenols," which may be responsible for the drop in blood pressure seen in the research. Not all extra-virgin olive oils are the same.[8]

I recommend organic, cold-pressed extra-virgin olive oil in dark glass bottles. Since olive oil can turn rancid, it needs to be kept in a dark pantry away from sunlight. Do not purchase huge bottles of olive oil in clear plastic bottles; you will not get the tremendous health benefits. Do not decrease your high blood pressure medication without first consulting with your doctor.

DARK CHOCOLATE

A potent antioxidant, dark chocolate contains plant phenols—cocoa phenols, to be exact—that are known to lower blood pressure.[9] A report published by Cochrane Collaborations that analyzed twenty studies found that people who eat a bit of dark chocolate or cocoa daily experienced a slight reduction in blood pressure. On average, the researchers discovered that flavonol-rich chocolate or cocoa powder reduced blood pressure on average by 2-3 mmHg. When antioxidants called flavonols that are found in chocolate are consumed, the body produces a substance called nitric oxide, according to the researchers. The chemical "relaxes" blood vessel walls, allowing blood to pass through with less obstruction.[10]

I often recommend some chocolates with high cocoa content (70 percent or higher) to patients with high blood pressure who have been instructed to lower their salt and carbohydrate intake. I also recommend dark chocolate low in sugar and with no dairy or trans fats.

POMEGRANATE

One of the most amazing foods when it comes to helping protect the heart is the pomegranate. The pomegranate has unique properties allowing it to help protect the inner lining of the arteries from damage. More and more research is showing pomegranate may even have the ability to reverse atherosclerosis (or hardening of the arteries from plaque buildup). I recommend 1 to 2 ounces of quality pomegranate juice two times per day. Supplements are also available.

One research study suggests that drinking 50 milliliters of pomegranate juice daily for up to a year can lower systolic blood pressure (the top number) by 5 to 21 percent. But drinking pomegranate juice doesn't seem to affect diastolic pressure (the lower number).[11]

In preliminary laboratory research and clinical trials, juice of the pomegranate may be effective in reducing heart disease risk factors, including LDL oxidation, macrophage oxidative status, and foam cell formation.[12] In mice, "oxidation of LDL by peritoneal macrophages was reduced by up to 90 percent after pomegranate juice consumption."[13]

Pomegranate contains a high amount of antioxidants called polyphenols, to which most of the fruit's benefits are attributed

One of the ways pomegranate might lower your blood pressure is by inhibiting angiotensin-converting enzyme activity, or ACE, according to a study conducted by researchers at the Rappaport Family Institute for Research in the Medical Sciences in Israel.

According to a study reported in the September 2001 issue of

Atherosclerosis, researchers observed that patients with hypertension taking 50 milliliters of pomegranate juice daily for two weeks experienced decreases in ACE activity and reductions in systolic blood pressure.[14]

BLUEBERRIES

When it comes to harnessing the power of antioxidants, blueberries rank number one when compared to other fruits and vegetables. Antioxidants help neutralize the damaging effects of free radicals that can lead to numerous diseases including heart disease, cancer, and Alzheimer's. Specific to the heart, the antioxidants in blueberries work to help reduce your cholesterol, decreasing your risk for heart attack and stroke. I recommend ¼–½ cup of organic fresh or frozen blueberries every day.

WILD SALMON

Oily fish such as salmon contain beneficial amounts of omega-3 fatty acids, or "good fat." Omega-3 fatty acids help reduce your level of triglycerides. Triglycerides are "bad fats" in the blood, increasing your risk of heart disease. Omega-3s also help keep the blood thin, reducing the risk of clots from sticking to arterial walls, a primary cause of fatal heart attacks. Omega-3s also help reduce the occurrence of dangerous heart arrhythmias, and they decrease inflammation in the body. The American Heart Association recommends eating 3 to 6 ounces of oily fish at least twice per week. I also recommend a good quality fish oil supplement as well. When it comes to fish, it is very important to make sure it is wild and low in mercury. (See Appendix B for fish low in mercury.) Steer away from farmed fish.

SPINACH

Dark, leafy green vegetables such as spinach, kale, swiss chard, and collards offer high levels of heart-healthy vitamins, minerals, and antioxidants. Similar to the nutrients in blueberries, these nutrients help reduce your risk of heart disease. Spinach in particular is also high in folate. Folate helps reduce homocysteine, a toxic amino acid that accelerates plaque formation and is usually a by-product from consuming meat. When homocysteine is present in high levels in the blood, it is associated with hardening and narrowing of the arteries, increased risk of heart attack, stroke, and blood clots. I recommend at least 1 cup a day of dark, leafy green vegetables a day.

WALNUTS

While nuts in general are a beneficial part of a healthy diet, walnuts contain almost twice the antioxidants as other nuts. Walnuts also contain high amounts of alpha-linolenic acid (ALA), which is associated with lower risk of heart attacks and blood clots. Nutrients in walnuts are also known for their vascular reactivity, or the ability of blood vessels to respond positively to changes in the environment.

Other heart-healthy superfoods deserving honorable mention include black beans, kidney beans, tomatoes, citrus fruits, oatmeal, cinnamon, green tea, and flaxseed.

MERCURY LEVELS IN FOOD

Lᴛʜᴏᴜɢʜ ғɪsʜ ɪs generally a good protein choice, some fish contain high levels of mercury. The following list will help you determine which fish to eat more liberally and which to avoid.[1]

Fish with least amounts of mercury (enjoy these fish)

- Anchovies
- Catfish
- Crab
- Flounder
- Haddock (Atlantic)
- Herring
- Salmon (fresh or canned)
- Sardines
- Shrimp
- Sole
- Tilapia
- Trout (freshwater)
- Whitefish

Fish with moderate amounts of mercury (eat six servings or less per month)

- Bass (striped or black)
- Halibut (Atlantic or Pacific)
- Lobster
- Mahi-Mahi
- Monkfish
- Snapper
- Tuna (canned, chunk light)

Fish high in mercury (eat three servings or less per month)

- Bluefish
- Grouper
- Mackerel (Spanish and Gulf)
- Sea bass (Chilean)
- Tuna (canned albacore)
- Tuna (yellowfin)

Fish highest in mercury (avoid)

- Mackerel (king)
- Marlin
- Orange roughy
- Shark
- Swordfish
- Tilefish
- Tuna (bigeye and ahi)

Appendix C

SUPPLEMENTS FOR WEIGHT LOSS AND REDUCING HYPERTENSION

M OST OF THE products mentioned throughout this book are offered through Dr. Colbert's Divine Health Wellness Center or are available at your local health food store.

Divine Health Nutritional Products
1908 Boothe Circle
Longwood, FL 32750
Phone: (407) 331-7007
Web site: www.drcolbert.com
E-mail: info@drcolbert.com

Maintenance nutritional supplements
- Divine Health Active Multivitamin
- Divine Health Living Multivitamin
- Divine Health Green Supreme Food

Omega oils
- Divine Health Living Omega

Protein powders
- Divine Health Plant Protein
- Divine Health Living Protein

Supplements for weight loss
- Fat Loss Drops

- PGX fiber
- Living Green Tea with EGCG
- Living Green Coffee Bean
- Meratrim (Metabolic Lean)
- MBS 360: contains green coffee bean and green tea with EGCG and Irvingia (available at www .mbs360.tv) This contains three fat-burners in one pill.
- 7-keto-DHEA

Supplements for thyroid support
- Metabolic Advantage
- Iodine Synergy

To curb food cravings
- Serotonin Max
- N-acetyl-tyrosine
- 5-HTP

Supplements to boost energy
- Divine Health Adrenal Support
- Divine Health PQQ
- Cellgevity (supplement to quench inflammation)

Supplements to lower high blood pressure
- Living CoQ_{10}
- Living nitric oxide
- L-arginine
- Watermelon seed
- Beet juice powder (Caution: may turn urine and/ or stool red.)

NOTES

INTRODUCTION
DISCOVER STRENGTH TO DEFEAT HIGH BLOOD PRESSURE

1. Centers for Disease Control and Prevention, "Vital Signs: Prevalence, Treatment, and Control of Hypertension—United States," 1999-2002 and 2005-2008, *MMWR.* 2011;60(4):103-8.
2. Ibid.
3. Ibid.
4. National Institute of Neurological Disorders and Stroke, "Stroke: Hope Through Research," National Institute on Health," http://www.ninds.nih.gov/disorders/stroke/detail_stroke.htm (accessed April 12, 2013).

1—UNDERSTANDING HIGH BLOOD PRESSURE

1. U.S. Department of Health and Human Services, "Reference Card From the Seventh Report of the Joint National Committee on Prevention, Detection, Evaluation, and Treatment of High Blood Pressure," May 2003, http://www.nhlbi.nih.gov/guidelines/hypertension/phycard.pdf (accessed March 7, 2013).
2. H. Klar Yaggi, John Concato, Walter N. Kernan, et al., "Obstructive Sleep Apnea as a Risk Factor for Stroke and Death," *New England Journal of Medicine* 353, no. 19 (November 10, 2005): 2034–2041, http://www.nejm.org/doi/full/10.1056/NEJMoa043104 (accessed May 23, 2013).
3. WebMD.com, "Causes of High Blood Pressure," http://www.webmd.com/hypertension-high-blood-pressure/guide/blood-pressure-causes (accessed May 24, 2013).

2—A HYPERTENSION-BUSTING DIET

1. Hypertension Institute of Nashville, "Nutritional Services: The DASH 1&2 Diet," http://www.hypertensioninstitute.com/dash-1-2.php (accessed May 23, 2013).
2. WebMD, "Salt Shockers Slideshow: High-Sodium Surprises." http://www.webmd.com/diet/ss/slideshow-salt-shockers (accessed May 9, 2013)
3. DASHDiet.org, "The DASH Diet Eating Plan," http://dashdiet.org/ (accessed April 3, 2013).
4. Ibid.
5. Ibid.

3—GET YOUR HEART IN SHAPE

1. TMZ.com, "Janet in Shape and in 'Control,'" July 27, 2006, http://www.tmz .com/2006/07/17/janet-in-shape-and-in-control/ (accessed April 12, 2013).

2. Rob Carnevale, "Bruce Willis: Die Hard 4.0," BBC, July 2, 2007, http:// www.bbc.co.uk/films/2007/07/02/bruce_willis_die_hard_4_2007_interview .shtml (accessed April 12, 2013).

3. Starpulse.com, "Memorable Celebrity Quotes," January 16, 2008, http:// www.starpulse.com/news/index.php/2008/01/16/memorable_celebrity_ quotes_118 (accessed April 12, 2013).

4. Mirelle Agaman, "Exclusive: Serena Williams Talks to Star!," *Star*, May 4, 2007.

5. Stephen Miller, "Jack LaLanne, Media Fitness Guru, Dies at 96," *Wall Street Journal*, January 24, 2011, http://online.wsj.com/article/SB100014240527487 03398504576100923135057068.html (accessed April 12, 2013).

6. Centers for Disease Control and Prevention (CDC), "Physical Activity and Health," http://www.cdc.gov/nccdphp/sgr/summ.htm (accessed April 12, 2013).

7. Jacqueline Stenson, "Excuses, Excuses," MSNBC.com, December 16, 2004, http://www.msnbc.msn.com/id/6391079/ns/health-fitness/t/excuses-excuses/ (accessed April 12, 2013).

8. Daniel J. DeNoon, "Chiropractic Cuts Blood Pressure," WebMD.com, http:// www.webmd.com/hypertension-high-blood-pressure/news/20070316/chiro- practic-cuts-blood-pressure (accessed May 23, 2013).

9. Centers for Disease Control and Prevention, "How Much Physical Activity Do Adults Need?", http://www.cdc.gov/physicalactivity/everyone/guidelines/ adults.html (accessed April 15, 2013).

10. Jennifer Corbett Dooren, "New Exercise Goal: 60 Minutes a Day," *Wall Street Journal*, March 24, 2010, http://online.wsj.com/article/SB1000142405 27487048961045751400111482664 70.html (accessed April 15, 2013).

11. Centers for Disease Control and Prevention, "How Much Physical Activity Do Adults Need?"

12. Peter Jaret, "A Healthy Mix of Rest and Motion," *New York Times*, May 3, 2007, http://tinyurl.com/c7zxot3 (accessed April 15, 2013).

13. K. N. Boutelle and D. S. Kirschenbaum, "Further Support for Consistent Self-Monitoring as a Vital Component of Successful Weight Control," *Obesity Research* 6, no. 3 (May 1998): 219–224, http://www.ncbi.nlm.nih .gov/pubmed/9618126 (accessed April 15, 2013).

4—FORTIFY YOUR HEART AND BLOOD VESSELS THROUGH SUPPLEMENTS

1. Brindusa Vanta, "Co-Enzyme Q-10 and Hypertention," LiveStrong.com, http://www.livestrong.com/article/318041-co-enzyme-q-10-and-hypertension/ (accessed May 9, 2013).

2. Peter Mitchell, "Uses of Olive Leaf Supplements," LiveStrong.com, http:// www.livestrong.com/article/520644-uses-of-olive-leaf-supplements/ (accessed May 9, 2013).

3. Michael Downey, "Olive Leaf Safely Modulates Blood Pressure," *Life Extension* magazine, March 2012, https://www.lef.org/magazine/mag2012/ mar2012_Olive-Leaf-Safely-Modulates-Blood-Pressure_01.htm (accessed May 9, 2013).

4. Bastyr Center for Natural Health, "Hibiscus Tea to Lower Your Blood Pressure," http://bastyrcenter.org/content/view/489/ (accessed May 9, 2013).

5. Herbs2000.com, "Chrysanthemum," http://www.herbs2000.com/herbs/ herbs_chrysanthemum.htm (accessed May 9, 2013).

6. *Forbes*, "Drinking Beetroot Juice Every Day Can Help Lower Blood Pressure by 7 Percent," http://www.forbes.com/sites/nadiaarumugam/2013/04/25/ drinking-beetroot-juice-every-day-can-help-lower-blood-pressure-by-7-percent/ (accessed May 9, 2013).

7. DoctorOz.com, "Alternative Health Trends for 2012," http://www.doctoroz .com/videos/alternative-health-trends-2012?page=3 (accessed May 9, 2013).

8. LifeExtension, "Three Foods That Lower High Blood Pressure," http://blog .lef.org/2009/09/three-foods-that-lower-high-blood.html (accessed May 9, 2013).

9. F. C. Luft and M. H. Weinberger, "Sodium Intake and Essential Hypertension," *Hypertension* 4, no. 5 (September–October 1982): 14–19.

10. One Life USA, "Melatonin Lowers Blood Pressure," http://onelifeusa.com/ health_news/Sleep%20Aids%2001.htm (accessed May 23, 2013); F. A. Scheer, G. A. Van Montfrans, E. J. van Someren, et al., "Daily Nighttime Melatonin Reduces Blood Pressure in Male Patients With Essential Hypertension," *Hypertension* 43, no. 2 (February 2004): 192–197.

5—YOUR HEART AND STRESS

1. Hans Selye, *The Stress of Life* (New York: McGraw-Hill, 1956).
2. Tara Parker-Pope, "The Secrets of Successful Aging," *Wall Street Journal*, http://online.wsj.com/article/0,,SB111867751964458052,00.html (accessed April 15, 2013).
3. D. A. Snowdon et al., "Linguistic Ability in Early Life and Cognitive Function and Alzheimer's Disease in Late Life. Findings From the Nun Study," *Journal of the American Medical Association* 275 (February 21, 1996): 528–532.
4. H. J. Eysenck et al., "Personality Type, Smoking Habit, and Their Interaction as Predictors of Cancer and Coronary Disease," *Personality and Individual Difference* 9, no.2 (1988): 479–495.
5. Ibid.
6. Ibid.
7. P. M. Plotsky et al., "PsychoNeural Endocrinology of Depression: Hypothalamic-Pituitary-Adrenal Axis," *Psychoneurology* 21, no. 2 (1998): 293–306.

6—COMBAT MODERN STRESS AT THE ROOT

1. T. Pickering, "Tension and Hypertension," *Journal of the American Medical Association* 370 (1993): 2494.
2. Richard A. Swenson, *The Overload Syndrome* (Colorado Springs, CO: NavPress, 1998).
3. Norman Cousins, *Anatomy of an Illness As Perceived by the Patient* (New York: Bantam, 1981).
4. Plotsky, "PsychoNeural Endocrinology of Depression: Hypothalamic-Pituitary-Adrenal Axis."

APPENDIX A: SUPERFOODS FOR YOUR HEART

1. Adapted from "Superfoods for Your Heart," DrColbert.com, March 14, 2013, http://www.drcolbert.com/blog/?p=146 (accessed April 9, 2013).
2. The World's Healthiest Foods, "Celery: What's New and Beneficial About Celery," WHFoods.com, http://www.whfoods.com/genpage.php?tname=foodspice&dbid=14 (accessed April 9, 2013).

3. Anne Hart, "Can Celery Really Lower Your Blood Pressure and Starve Cancer Cells?", Examiner.com, http://www.examiner.com/article/can-celery -really-lower-your-blood-pressure-and-starve-cancer-cells (accessed May 9, 2013).

4. Kathleen M. Zelman, "The Truth About Beetroot Juice," WebMD.com, http://www.webmd.com/food-recipes/features/truth-about-beetroot-juice (accessed April 9, 2013).

5. *Forbes*, "Drinking Beetroot Juice Every Day Can Help Lower Blood Pressure by 7 Percent."

6. F. G. McMahon and R. Vargas, "Can Garlic Lower Blood Pressure? A Pilot Study," *Pharmacotherapy* 13, no. 4 (July–August 1993): 406–407, http://www.ncbi.nlm.nih.gov/pubmed/8361870; WebMD, "Find a Vitamin or Supplement: Garlic," http://tinyurl.com/8654woj (accessed May 9, 2013).

7. Donald Hensrud, "If Olive Oil Is High in Fat, Why Is It Considered Healthy?" MayoClinic.com, http://www.mayoclinic.com/health/food-and -nutrition/AN01037 (accessed April 9, 2013).

8. Elizabeth Tracy, "Extra-Virgin Olive Oil Reduces Need for Blood Pressure Medication," WebMD.com, http://tinyurl.com/d6a9xwp (accessed May 9, 2013).

9. Daniel J. DeNoon, "Dark Chocolate Is Healthy Chocolate," WebMD.com, August 27, 2003, http://www.webmd.com/diet/news/20030827/dark-chocolate-is-healthy-chocolate (accessed April 9, 2013).

10. Michelle Castillo, "Flavonol-Rich Dark Chocolate May Help Reduce Blood Pressure," CBS News, http://www.cbsnews.com/8301-504763_162-57494718 -10391704/flavonol-rich-dark-chocolate-may-help-reduce-blood-pressure/ (accessed May 10, 2013).

11. MedlinePlus, "Pomegranate," http://www.nlm.nih.gov/medlineplus/druginfo/ natural/392.html (accessed May 9, 2013).

12. M. Aviram, M. Rosenblat, D. Gaitini, et al., "Pomegranate Juice Consumption for Three Years by Patients With Carotid Artery Stenosis Reduces Common Carotid Intima-Media Thickness, Blood Pressure and LDL Oxidation," *American Journal of Clinical Nutrition* 23, no. 3 (June 2004): 423–433; Ahmad Esmaillzadeh, Farideh Tahbaz, Iraj Gaieni, et al., "Concentrated Pomegranate Juice Improves Lipid Profiles in Diabetic Patients With Hyperlipidemia," *Journal of Medicinal Food* 7, no. 3 (Fall 2004): 305–308; Marielle Kaplan, Tony Hayek, Ayelet Raz, et al., "Pomegranate Juice Supplementation to Atherosclerotic Mice Reduces Macrophage Lipid Peroxidation, Cellular Cholesterol Accumulation and Development of Atherosclerosis," *Journal of Nutrition* 131, no. 8 (August 1, 2001): 2082–2089.

13. Michael Aviram, Leslie Dornfeld, Mira Rosenblat, et al., "Pomegranate Juice Consumption Reduces Oxidative Stress, Atherogenic Modifications to LDL, and Platelet Aggregation: Studies in Humans and in Atherosclerotic Apolipoprotein E-Deficient Mice," *American Journal of Clinical Nutrition* 71, no. 5 (May 2000): 1062–1076.

14. Brandon Dotson, "Does Pomegranate Lower Blood Pressure?", Livestrong .com, http://www.livestrong.com/article/469377-does-pomegranate-lower -blood-pressure/ (accessed May 9, 2013).

APPENDIX B: MERCURY LEVELS IN FOOD

1. "Mercury Contamination in Fish: A Guide to Staying Healthy and Fighting Back," Natural Resources Defense Council, http://www.nrdc.org/health/ effects/mercury/guide.asp (accessed May 24, 2013).

Don Colbert, MD, was born in Tupelo, Mississippi. He attended Oral Roberts School of Medicine in Tulsa, Oklahoma, where he received a bachelor of science degree in biology in addition to his degree in medicine. Dr. Colbert completed his internship and residency with Florida Hospital in Orlando, Florida. He is board certified in family practice and anti-aging medicine and has received extensive training in nutritional medicine.

If you would like more
information about natural and
divine healing, or information about
Divine Health nutritional products,
you may contact Dr. Colbert at:

Don Colbert, MD
1908 Boothe Circle
Longwood, FL 32750
Telephone: 407-331-7007 (for ordering products only)
Website: www.drcolbert.com.

Disclaimer: Dr. Colbert and the staff of Divine Health Wellness Center are prohibited from addressing a patient's medical condition by phone, facsimile, or e-mail. Please refer questions related to your medical condition to your own primary care physician.

Pick up these great Bible Cure books by Don Colbert, MD:

TAKE CONTROL OF **YOUR HEALTH**
THE NATURAL WAY

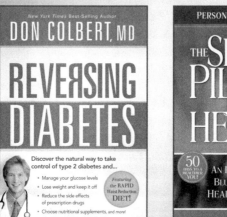

978-1-61638-598-9 | US $16.99

REVERSING DIABETES
Learn to manage and even
reverse type 2 diabetes naturally

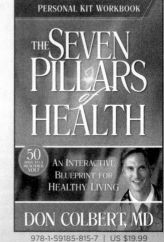

978-1-59185-815-7 | US $19.99

THE SEVEN PILLARS OF HEALTH
A *New York Times* best seller!
Restore your health and reclaim
your life with this fifty-day,
biblically based plan.

AVAILABLE EVERYWHERE
BOOKS ARE SOLD